Prosthesis

Edited by Ramana Vinjamuri

Published in London, United Kingdom

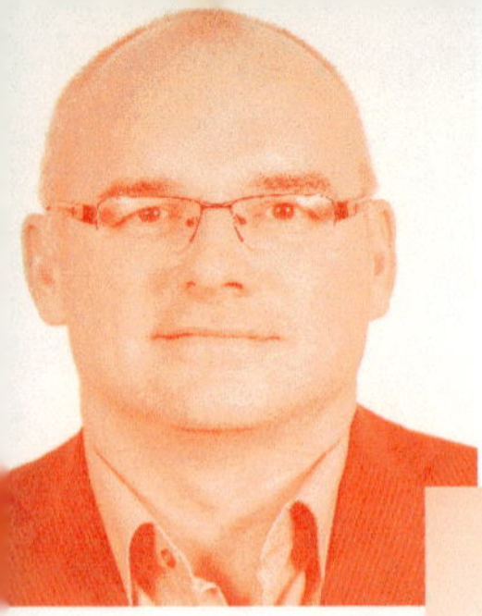
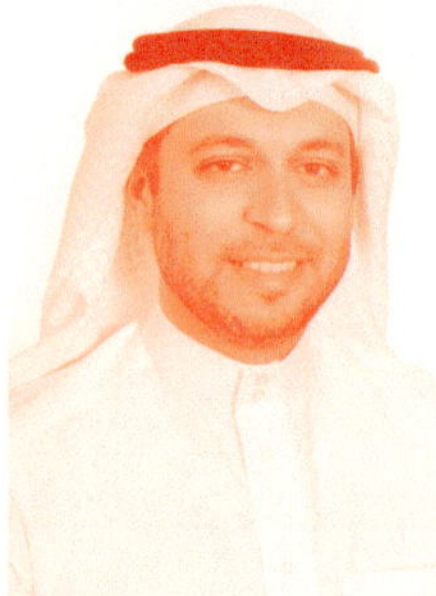
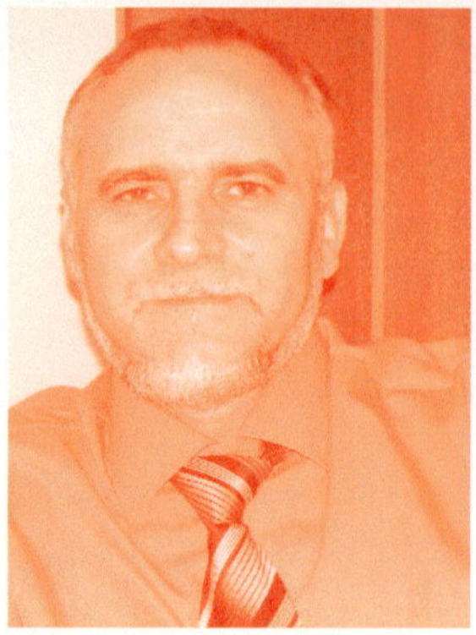
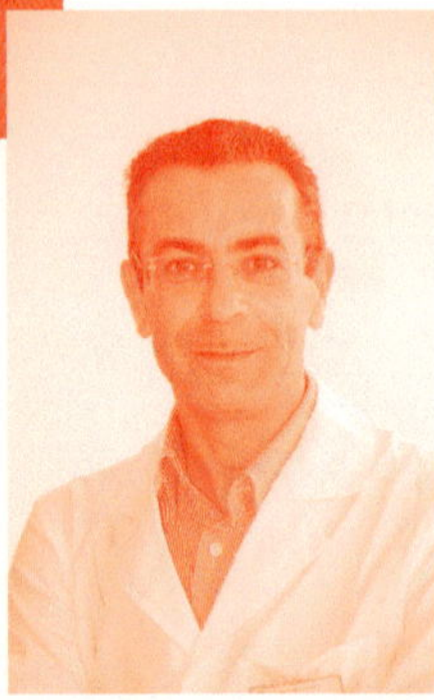
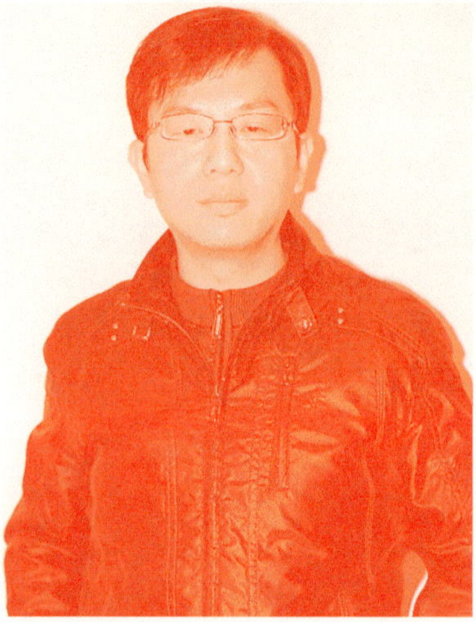
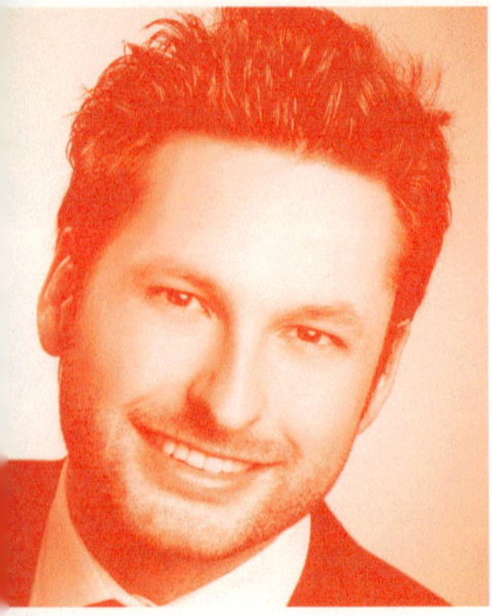
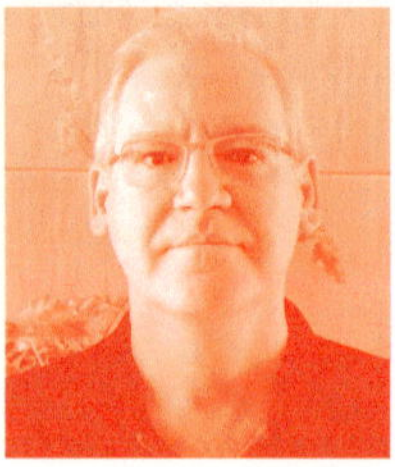

IntechOpen

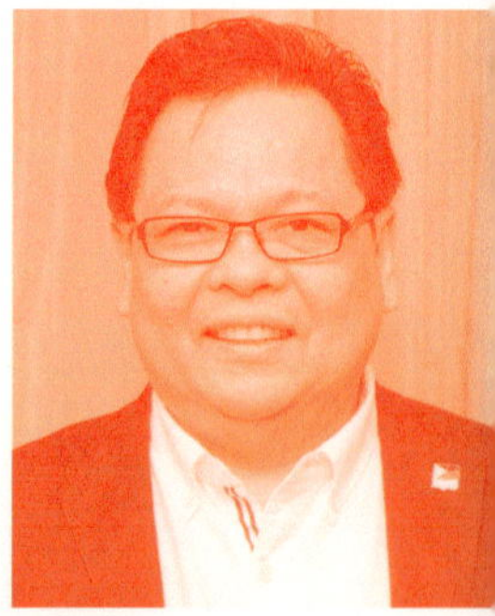
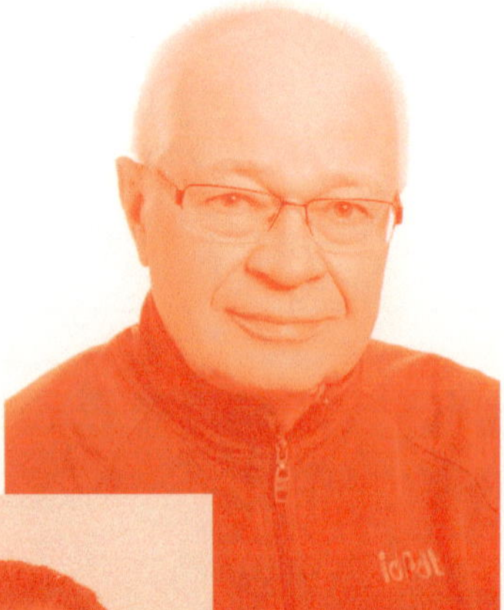
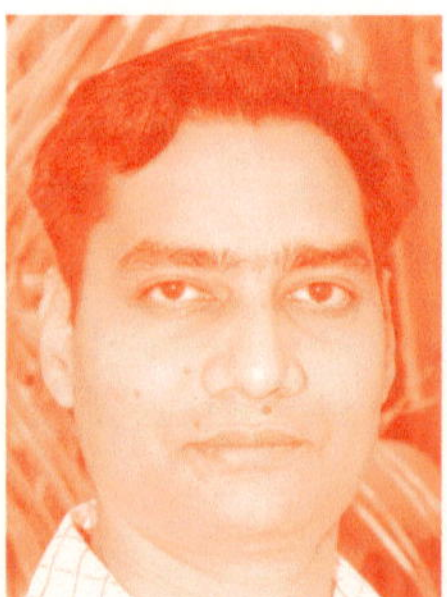
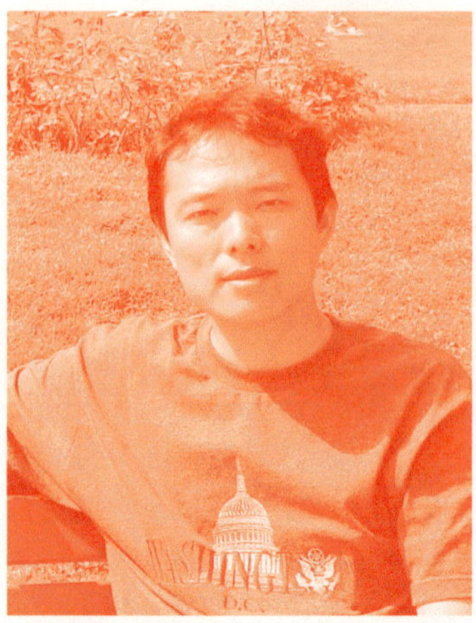
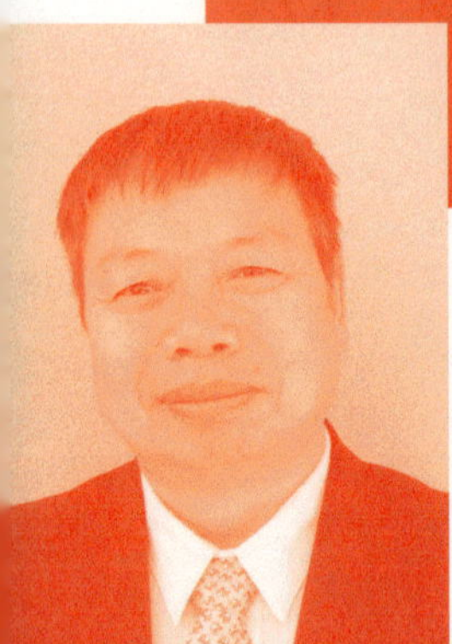
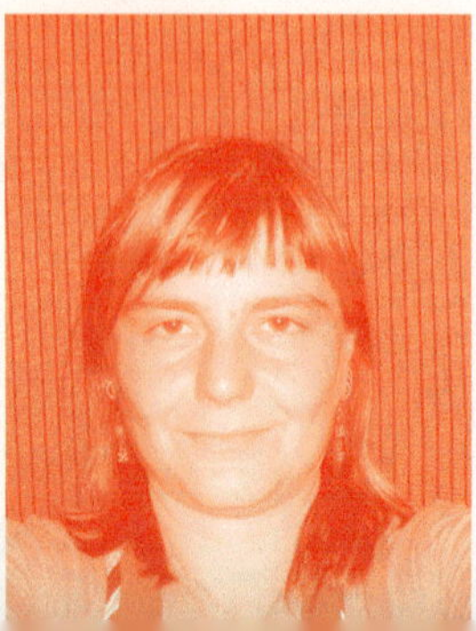

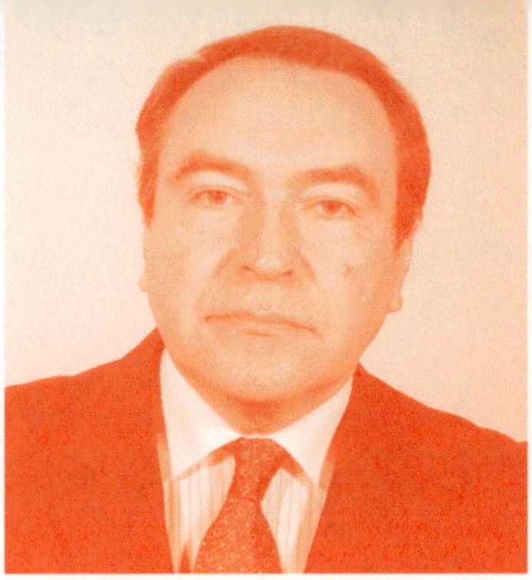
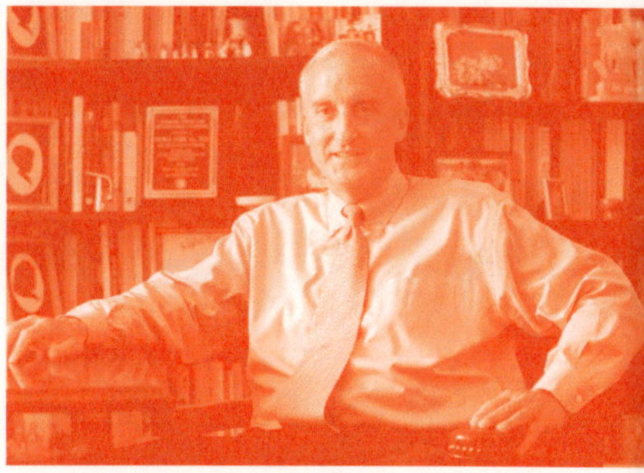
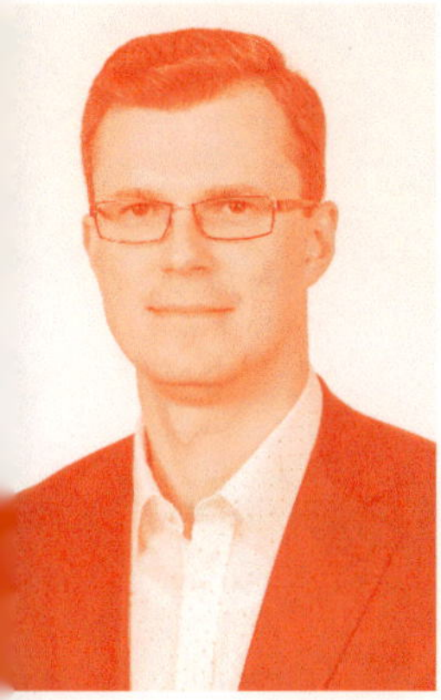
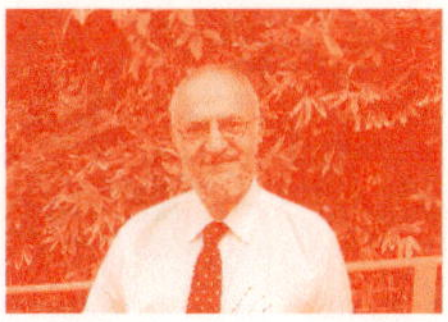
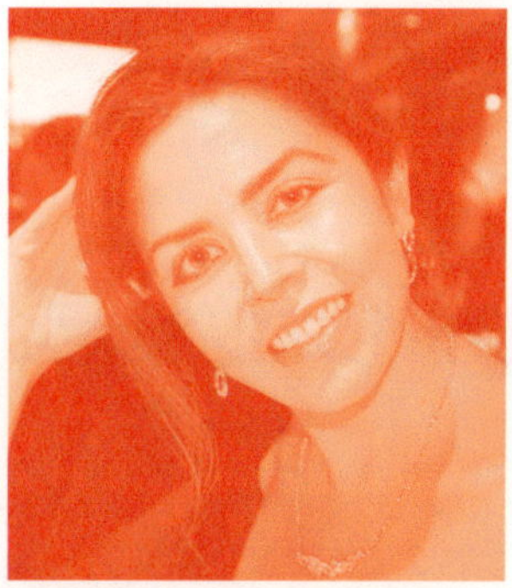

Supporting open minds since 2005

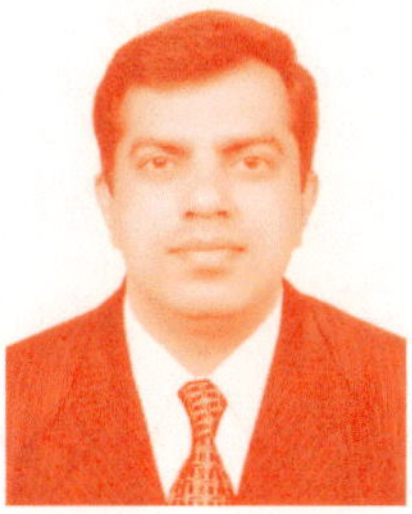
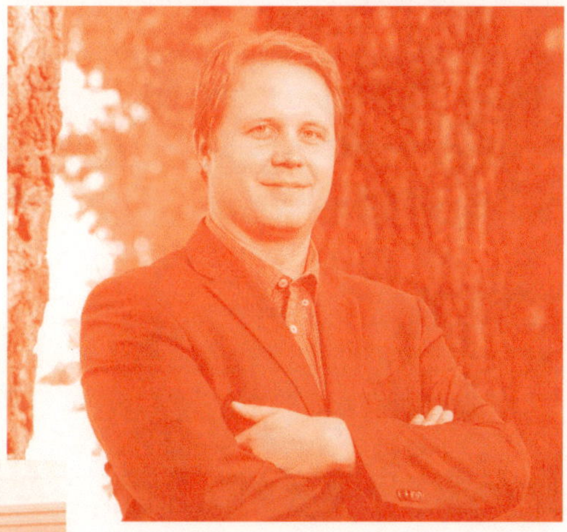
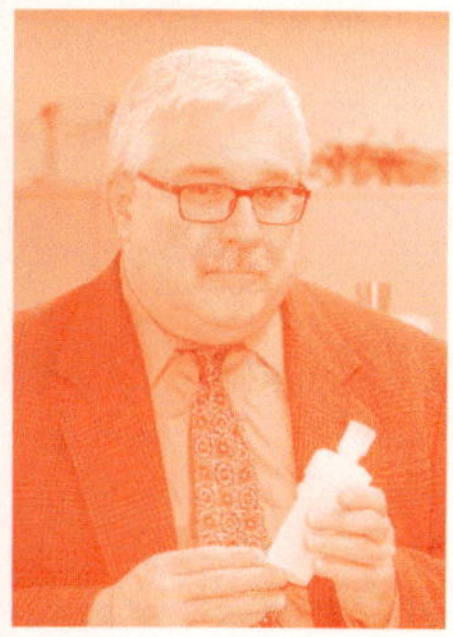
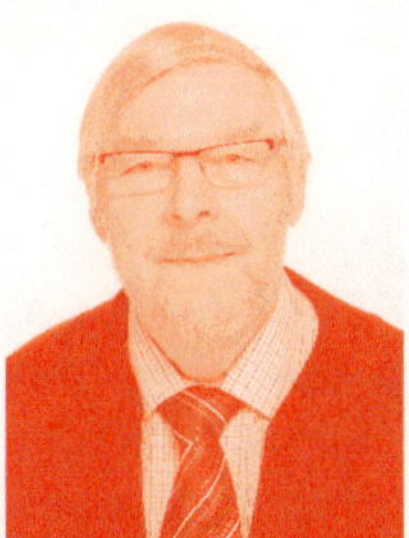
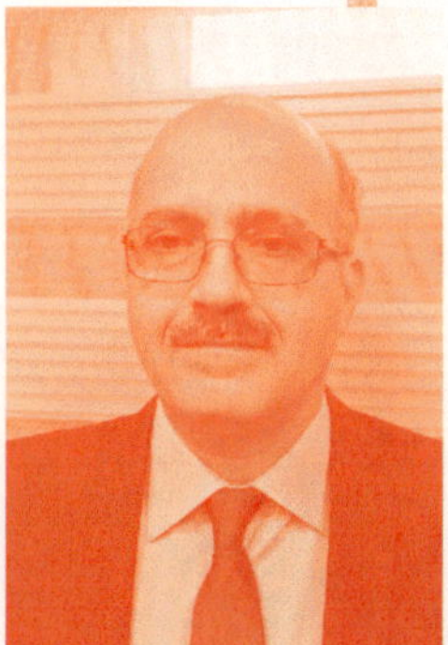
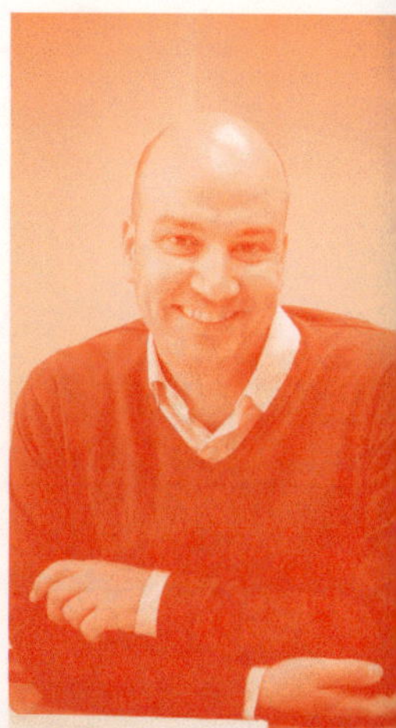
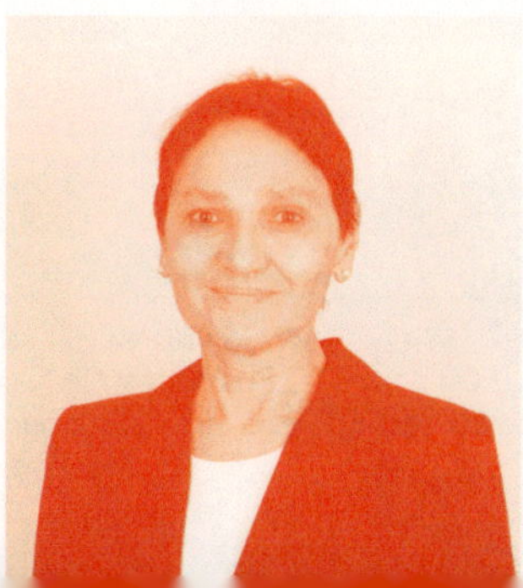

Prosthesis
http://dx.doi.org/10.5772/intechopen.73978
Edited by Ramana Vinjamuri

Contributors
Daniel Odebiyi, Caleb Adewumi Adeagbo, Chandan K Sen, Sashwati Roy, Shomita Mathew-Steiner, Percy Nohama, Guilherme Nogueira Neto, Maira Ranciaro, Edward Bloch, Lyndon Da Cruz, Faraedon M. Mostafa, Kaida Xiao, Yohei Muraguchi, Wenwei Yu, Ramana Vinjamuri

First published in London, United Kingdom, 2020 by IntechOpen
IntechOpen is the global imprint of INTECHOPEN LIMITED, registered in England and Wales, registration number: 11086078, 7th floor, 10 Lower Thames Street, London, EC3R 6AF, United Kingdom
Printed in Croatia

British Library Cataloguing-in-Publication Data
A catalogue record for this book is available from the British Library

Additional hard and PDF copies can be obtained from orders@intechopen.com

Prosthesis
Edited by Ramana Vinjamuri
p. cm.
Print ISBN 978-1-83880-153-3
Online ISBN 978-1-83880-381-0
eBook (PDF) ISBN 978-1-83880-382-7

For EU product safety concerns:
IN TECH d.o.o., Prolaz Marije Krucifikse Kozulić 3, 51000 Rijeka, Croatia, info@intechopen.com or visit our website at intechopen.com.

Meet the editor

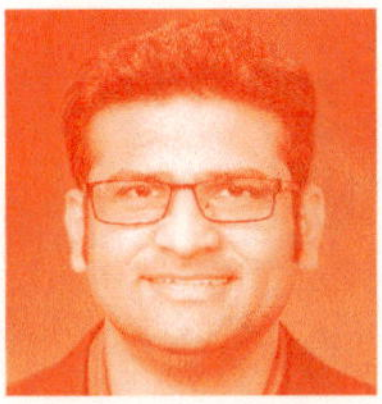

Ramana Vinjamuri received his undergraduate degree in Electrical Engineering from Kakatiya University (India) in 2002. He received his MS in Electrical Engineering from Villanova University in 2004, specializing in Bioinstrumentation. He received his PhD in Electrical Engineering in 2008 specializing in Dimensionality Reduction in Control and Coordination of Human Hand from the University of Pittsburgh. He has worked as a postdoctoral fellow (2008-2012) in the field of Brain Machine Interfaces (BMI) to control prostheses in the School of Medicine, University of Pittsburgh. He has worked as a Research Assistant Professor in the Department of Biomedical Engineering at the Johns Hopkins University (2012-2013). He is currently a Harvey N Davis Distinguished Assistant Professor in the Department of Biomedical Engineering at the Stevens Institute of Technology. He received the NSF CAREER Award in 2019. He also holds a secondary appointment as an Adjunct Assistant Professor at the Indian Institute of Technology, Hyderabad, India.

Contents

Preface

In February 2018, my first book titled "Biomimetic Prosthetics" was published by IntechOpen. This was an edited volume with contributions from researchers all over the world on biomimetic (mimicking complex biological sensorimotor systems of human beings and animals) prosthetics. With over 2500 downloads, multiple citations and compliments from my colleagues, this was a rewarding experience. I would like to thank the authors for their valuable contributions and staff at IntechOpen in this book project. I would also like to extend my special thanks to my students from the Sensorimotor Control Laboratory at Stevens who contributed towards the introductory chapter of this book. In June 2018, I was approached by commissioning editors at IntechOpen to see if I was interested in leading another edited volume on "Prostheses". This could cover a broader category of prostheses and appeal to a wider audience. I took some time and responded favorably for the following reason. During my previous project on Biomimetic Prosthetics, I rejected several applications on prosthetics as they were not necessarily biomimetic. During that project I realized that there was a need to provide another opportunity for these other valuable contributions. This came to me in the form of this current book "Prosthesis". It has been a great learning experience and an inspiring academic journey through these book projects.

In this book, the readers will find information on various prostheses for upper limb, lower limb, retinal, and facial prostheses. These areas of research are multidisciplinary, requiring expertise in electrical engineering, mechanical engineering, biomedical engineering, material sciences, and tissue engineering. The uniqueness of the field of prostheses is in combining multiple expertise to improve technologies that can help individuals with impairments.

The introductory chapter presents the evolution of prosthesis and their applications in different domains. This chapter prepares the readers with the context, application, and importance of prosthesis.

The second chapter talks about control methods for the transhumeral prosthesis considering the task environment and object properties. Specifically, this study explores how using such information coupled with around-shoulder muscle action potentials targeted reaching positions that can be accurately and rapidly identified.

While the second chapter talks about upper limb prosthesis and control, the third chapter talks about hybrid neuroprosthesis for lower limbs. This chapter summarizes the principles of human mobility and the impact of spinal cord injury on an individual's mobility. This chapter also talks about how a hybrid prosthesis combined with functional electric stimulation and orthoses can be used to reactivate paralyzed muscles and enable function.

In the fourth chapter, residual lower limb health and possible prosthetics are discussed. Changes in residual limb properties may affect socket fit and may lead to serious injuries. This chapter presents socket systems available in the market and compares them with the elevated vacuum suspension system that could improve and provide physiological benefits to the residual limb.

In the fifth chapter, ambulatory assistive devices for individuals with injuries or disabilities in lower extremities are discussed. These devices play an important role in providing support, stability, and balance. In particular, this chapter talks about some useful guidelines in prescriptive ambulatory devices.

Switching gears to other prosthesis systems, the next two chapters talk about retinal prosthesis and facial prosthesis. In the sixth chapter, an overview is given of the Argus II retinal prosthesis system, as well as requirements, results achieved to date, challenges, and some future directions.

In the seventh chapter, using additive manufacturing, 3D color printed soft tissue facial prostheses are described. The chapter talks in detail about methods involved in assessing mechanical properties of materials, infiltrating them with silicone polymers, and testing their specifications for their potential use for facial prosthesis.

This book is a representative compilation of several types of prostheses, their importance, their challenges, and recent scientific and technological developments. I would like to thank the authors with diverse expertise for their valuable contributions. I would also like to thank IntechOpen staff especially Josip Knapic, Petra Svob, and Martina Brkljacic for their kind assistance throughout the editing process. Without their help, this book would just remain an idea. I hope that the readers will be informed and inspired from reading this book.

Ramana Vinjamuri and Harvey N Davis
Distinguished Assistant Professor,
Director of Sensorimotor Control Laboratory,
Department of Biomedical Engineering,
Schaefer School of Engineering,
Stevens Institute of Technology,
New Jersey, USA

Chapter 1

Introductory Chapter: Past, Present, and Future of Prostheses and Rehabilitation

Shanthini Madhanagopal, Martin Burns, Dingyi Pei, Rohan Mukundhan, Helen Meyerson and Ramana Vinjamuri

1. Background

A prosthesis is defined as "...a device attached to the stump of an amputated body part due to traumatic or congenital conditions..." [1]. Prostheses have evolved over the past centuries, starting with a wooden toe to the highly mechanized robotic limbs of today. The evolution of prosthesis started in the Egyptian period during which wood was used as a replacement for a missing toe, coconut shell was used as a dental implant, and various other materials were used as an alternative to different body parts. There are various types of prostheses depending on the body part being replaced. These include upper and lower limb (LL) prostheses, neural prostheses (NP), retinal prostheses, maxillofacial prostheses, and various other types. Each prosthesis is designed and assembled based on the person's physical appearance, functional needs, and affordability [2–7]. The history of lower limb prosthesis is outlined in **Table 1**. This is a summary of our findings from [8, 9].

Amputations are estimated to occur between 300 and 500 times per day, leading to an increased usage of prostheses [10]. With increased need there are various factors which impact prosthesis usage, including whether the amputation is unilateral or bilateral, the time duration between amputation and prosthetic fitting, type of prosthesis used, physical health factors such as phantom-limb pain, and the psychological impact of amputation such as perception of symptoms, self-efficiency, balance confidence, treatment cost, and time taken to adapt to the prosthesis. The quality of life post-rehabilitation does not solely depend on the abovementioned factors but also includes functional utility and satisfaction over time. Improvements in quality of life are possible with recent innovations in design tools, materials, and different types of manufacturing, aiding in customizing prosthesis according to patient needs [11]. Novel rehabilitation methods, different types of prostheses, their limitations, and recent advancements will be discussed in this chapter.

2. Virtual reality rehabilitation

Upper limb (UL) paralysis and other motor deficits are common after a stroke. About 70% of acute phase patients and 50% of chronic phase patients experience such deficits. Upper limb paralysis affects tens of thousands worldwide, and all the forms of paralysis as a whole affect millions [12]. Currently, there is no way to safely cure paralysis. Instead, upper limb paralysis patients undergo rehabilitation treatment

IntechOpen

Year	Type of prosthetic	Material/technology
600 B.C	Below knee	Wooden peg leg
1500	Below knee	Esthetic iron leg
1600	Below knee	Armor-based sheet metal leg
1650	Below knee	Metal casting with leather straps
1696	Below knee	Wooden foot with copper socket
1800	Above knee with ischial seat	First hardened leather with knee joint
1816	Anglesey leg	First wood and steel-based joint articulating leg
1851	Benjamin Palmer leg	Spring with metal tendons
1863	Dubois L. Parmelee	Pressure-based limb and socket attachment
1865	Dollinger foot	Foot with rocking sole
1900	Bumper foot	Solid rubber foot
1912	Leg	Aluminum-based lightweight leg
1915	Leg	Metal leg with lifelike appearance
1920	Leg	Metal replaced wood to reduce weight
1950	Leg	First adjustable steel bar-based prosthesis
1990	Knee	First microprocessor knee
2009	Leg	Carbon fiber-based sprinter

Table 1.
Evolution of lower limb prostheses.

which gradually improves their lost function with exercises and stretches. There are many different approaches to provide treatment, which include working with a physical therapist on hand motor and strength skills and using prosthetic devices, such as robotic exoskeletons. The exoskeleton is a wearable, electrical device that straps onto the impaired arm or hand. It improves the limb's strength and endurance and its motor abilities by allowing the brain and the upper limb to regain communication [13].

In recent years, the use of virtual reality (VR) simulations designed in environments such as Unity has emerged to provide post-trauma and post-stroke rehabilitation. Hardware such as VR goggles and the Leap Motion controller, as well as Cybergloves and joysticks, are used to manipulate objects in virtual reality to provide an alternative to conventional rehabilitation methods. Improvements in retention and ease of use are accomplished by creating more immersive and engaging exercises for patients than the standard approach. Games with goals and challenges, interesting environments, and different types of in-game rewards can provide extra motivation to the patient. There has been a wide variety of studies researching the use of a virtual reality environment for rehabilitation of different impairments. In one study, VR rehabilitation for a 6-DoF ankle prosthetic was used to supplement robotic therapy. Subjects were put into an environment where they needed to navigate a plane or a boat; results showed that the VR group showed a larger increase in walking speed as well as higher retention rates and 28% less audiovisual cues needed during the experiment than those who used the robot alone [14]. Upper limb rehabilitation was also performed for subjects learning to use complex prostheses with multiple dimensions [15]. Games like MindBalance require the subject to control an animated character and balance checkerboards on a tightrope, with a "3 strikes" approach to balance. During a test, subjects achieved 89% accuracy due to the EEG-based BCI performance [16]. Patients who experienced upper-extremity (UE) deficits improved forearm extension and movement as well as hand-eye coordination, control and endurance of the UE, strength of the UE, and flexibility through VR [17].

As VR technology develops further, researchers must consider factors such as graphics design to maintain immersion without disorienting the patient. Elements from conventional rehabilitation known to promote good outcomes, such as task repetition [18], must also be incorporated into the design of the games. VR rehabilitation methods are becoming attractive alternatives to conventional physical/occupational therapy. They promise more efficient and less expensive therapies, increasing patient access and decreasing the amount of time necessary for rehabilitation.

3. Upper limb prosthesis

Upper limb prostheses are some of the most commonly used prosthetic devices since the human hand and arm is a vital tool for interaction, sensing, and working in an environment. Major limb amputations have been estimated to occur in 1 out of every 300 people in the United States, with 23% involving the upper extremity [19]. Unlike other types of amputation, most UL amputations are due to trauma. The evolution of UL prostheses has been exceptional over the past decades, resulting in highly mechanized devices which improve the quality of life of amputees by enabling them to perform activities of daily living (ADL).

UL prostheses can be classified based on the type of amputation and type of control mechanism. The type of amputation can be classified as trans-humeral, trans-radial, wrist, trans-metacarpal, and trans-phalangeal. Within these types, trans-radial is the most commonly used UL prostheses as it accounts for up to 10% of upper limb amputation [20]. Based on the type of control mechanism, these devices can be divided into body-powered, externally powered, and hybrid-controlled systems. Body-powered systems use body movements to control a terminal device or a joint like the elbow. Externally battery-powered systems use electric switches or myoelectric signals for control, activated by residual limb movements or electromyographic signals generated by the residual limb. Hybrid systems combine body and external power control to balance weight, cost, and cosmetics and accommodate different amputation levels.

Rejection rates for UL prostheses have been high, ranging from 3 to 60% in most studies with rates closer to 60%. This rate was shown to correlate to the proximity of amputation with 6% for trans-radial and 60% for shoulder disarticulation [20, 21]. Many studies show that amputees are not satisfied with their prosthetic, thus resulting in high abandonment rates. There are various factors which affect prosthetic usage, and there are a lot of discrepancies between the various studies. For example, a study conducted by Burger et al. in a group of 414 upper limb amputees showed that factors such as level of amputation, loss of dominant hand, and time between prosthesis fitting and amputation play an important role in prosthetic use [22]. Other studies consider factors related to demographic impacts such as education level, level of amputation acceptance, and economic factors such as prosthetic use and training expense. These can be collectively considered as psycho-economic factors [23]. Based on this, the factors being considered have to be better understood to know their actual impact on prosthetic use.

4. Lower limb prosthesis

Lower limb prostheses provide support and assist in locomotion for lower limb amputees. Lower limb prosthetics can assist many amputees to regain independence and mobility, thereby improving their quality of life. An estimate of 185,000 lower extremity amputations happens each year within the United States and may double by 2050. Unlike UL amputation, LL amputation is due to various reasons such as vascular diseases like diabetes, peripheral arterial disease, trauma, and cancer [24]. In the case of amputation related to vascular diseases, there is a likely chance that within the next few years, the other leg is also amputated. Diabetes is a major factor in the case of vascular-related amputation as it affects 8.3% of the US population with an incidence of 5.7 per 100,000 people [25]. Ninety percent of new amputations concern the lower extremity with 53% of patients requiring a transtibial amputation and 39% accounting for transfemoral amputation [26].

The main components of a lower limb prosthesis include the socket, suspension, knee unit (if required), foot/ankle complex, and any other components based on the patient's comfort level. LL prostheses can be classified into several different categories as transfemoral, transtibial, ankle, and foot-based devices. Each of these categories has its type of socket and suspension to improve contact and proper attachment. Types of transtibial socket designs include a patellar tendon bearing socket which uses the patellar ligament as a partial weight-bearing surface or a total surface bearing socket which distributes equal pressure on the stump. Transtibial suspension types include a supracondylar cuff, a lanyard system, a supracondylar suspension, or an older model which is a thigh corset with side joints. Transfemoral socket designs include quadrilateral and ischial containment. Suction is the most common form of a transfemoral suspension, with a pelvic band prescribed for some patients. Types of prosthetic knee include manual locking, which are single-axis knees with a single axis of rotation, hydraulics or pneumatic polycentric knees, and microprocessor-controlled knees. Microprocessor-controlled knees utilize a microprocessor to control the pneumatics or hydraulics throughout the gait cycle. Types of prosthetic foot include the solid ankle cushion heel (SACH), single-axis foot, multi-axis foot, and dynamic response feet. The latter have a flexible heel that stores potential energy during early stance phase that is then released through recoil of the material in the late stance and early swing phase. Partial foot prosthesis options include toe fillers with or without orthosis and shoe modifications [27].

LL prostheses can be categorized into three types of control mechanisms: passive, semi-active, and active. Passive devices perform like a fixed spring and damper and hence offer only basic functionality. Semi-active prostheses are capable of instantaneously altering movement, utilizing microprocessors to react to situations. They offer greater flexibility than passive devices but are limited to generating resistive forces. Active prostheses are externally powered by batteries and driven by motors regulating their movement. This gives active prostheses the ability to act instead of react without a lag compared to the former types. Thus they offer greater performance and functionality, but the overall system is highly complex and heavy [28]. While the different types of LL devices have their advantages, disadvantages, and constraints, these qualities are being overcome by technological innovations. New design tools and manufacturing techniques like 3D printing mitigate the constraints of the current state of the art and support in customizing prosthetics according to patient needs.

5. Neural prosthesis

The foremost intent of neural prostheses is to form an interface between a device and neural tissue to directly interact with the nervous system of individuals with neurological disorders like amyotrophic lateral sclerosis. This interface is known as the brain machine interface which is the core of NP and makes it feasible to study brain mechanisms. An estimation of 11,000 and 700,000 spinal cord injury and stroke cases has been reported per year, respectively, with an increasing need for NPs that can be utilized for sensory restoration to improve the quality of life of individuals [29]. An NP can either be an input device which converts surrounding information into perceptions, such as cochlear implants, or an output interface which converts the brain's intentions into activity. There are many types of neuroprosthetics that can be broadly classified as invasive or noninvasive. The former is more complicated since any fault with the device or the connection will require a revision surgery, which will impact the patient both physically and economically [30]. NPs include devices ranging from basic electrical stimulators to multichannel percutaneously implanted electrode systems.

NPs can be further classified into two types based on the type of stimulation, such as functional neuromuscular stimulation (FNS) or cerebellar stimulation. In FNS, electrical stimulation is used to activate or inhibit skeletal muscles based on the type of injury. FNS is used for various applications like lower and upper extremity rehabilitation, auditory prostheses, and respiratory disorders. In lower extremity rehabilitation, NPs were used to correct foot drop in stroke patients by stimulation of the peroneal nerve with resultant activation of the tibialis muscle during the swing phase of gait [29]. Upper extremity rehabilitation involves restoring the ability to elevate the shoulder, raise the upper arm, and flex the elbow in the presence of a paralyzed lower arm and hand. FNS-based NPs are used to treat sensory deafness if the hair cells are still intact with the brain to produce sensations of sound by electrically stimulating the fibers. Ondine's curse, a respiratory disorder caused by the lesion of upper motor neurons, results in the ineffective movement of the diaphragm which can be treated by stimulation of phrenic nerves. This is called FNS-based electrophrenic prosthesis and has replaced mechanical respirators. In the case of cerebellar stimulation, electrical current is passed through electrodes placed on the surface of the cerebellum. This technique is used as a treatment option for various conditions such as intractable epilepsy, multiple sclerosis, cerebral palsy, intention tremor, and many different types of motor disorders [29].

There are various limitations of NPs. First, the contact area between the sensory implant and the neural tissue is relatively small compared to anatomical neurons in the sensory pathway. Second, implants are placed in the sensory pathways that have been severed. With a lesion in this pathway, there is usually less chance of regeneration due to reduced interface with the electrode. Third, electrodes contacting the neural tissue are prone to rejection and degradation with a chance of potential damage to the stimulating neural tissue. Fourth, refractory properties limit the number of electrical impulses a neuron will respond to in a given time interval. Fifth, size, biocompatibility, durability, and energy supply are some of the basic problems with NPs [29]. Other factors include treatment cost, recovery, and handling. These problems become serious issues as a majority of stroke patients are elderly people who cannot withstand such intense operations and require more recovery time than young adults. Thus, with further advancements, the complexity of NP can also be reduced, thereby increasing its applications.

6. Retinal prostheses

The first visual prostheses were invented in the 1960s, demonstrating that visual perception of the subject can be restored by electrical stimulation of the visual cortex using 180 cortical surface electrodes [31]. In normal visual perception, light travels through various chambers of the eye including the cornea, aqueous humor, pupil, lens, and vitreous chamber to activate photoreceptors and set up the trans-synaptic connections of the retina [32]. Four important parts of the eye in visual perception are the lens, cornea, retina, and retinal pigmented epithelium. Any defect in one of these parts can cause blindness. Several intractable blinding conditions are due to retinal damage, the most common type being retinal degeneration. This can be broadly classified into two categories: photoreceptor rod degeneration like retinitis pigmentosa, and macular photoreceptor cone degeneration like age-related macular degeneration (AMD). The prevalence of rod degeneration is estimated to be about 1 in 3500 around the world. It is also estimated that 2 million Americans above the age of 55 have AMD, with another 7 million being pre-symptomatic [33]. Retinal prostheses try to reactivate the residual circuitry in a blind patient's retina to produce a synthetic form of usable vision. Using an array of stimulus electrodes or light-sensitive proteins, the neurons in the degenerate retinal network are activated to elicit a series of light percepts termed "phosphenes." This acts as independent spatial percepts in their visual field, restoring a crude form of vision [34].

The type of prosthesis is chosen based on the condition of the subject's vision. Different types of retinal prostheses include epiretinal prosthetics, in which the device is implanted into the vitreous cavity, and subretinal prosthetics, where the device is implanted in the potential space between the retinal pigment epithelium and neurosensory retina to stimulate the outer retina. Epiretinal prostheses like the Argus II include an imaging device like a camera which transforms visual information into patterns of electrical stimulation administered to viable retinal neurons. In the case of subretinal prosthesis, a micro-photodiode array (MPDA) is implanted between the retinal pigment epithelium and bipolar cell layer, which enhances vision in patients with RP and AMD. It can be considered as a replacement for lost photoreceptors [35].

Epiretinal and subretinal devices have their advantages and disadvantages. Advantages of subretinal devices include a lower current requirement and the lack of a need for mechanical fixation due to its proximity to the visual neurons. Disadvantages include the limited subretinal space and the increased risk of thermal damage to the neurons due to heat dissipation in the vitreous humor [36]. Advantages of epiretinal devices include reduced thermal damage to the neurons, a reduced number of electrodes, and a flexible procedure for subsequent surgeries. Disadvantages include increased electrical current requirements and adhesion of the device to the inner retina, which is more technically challenging [37].

7. Maxillofacial prostheses

A maxillofacial prosthesis is an artificial replacement for facial features to restore oral functions such as swallowing, mastication, and speech. There are numerous causes which can be congenital, traumatic, or disease-borne in nature. Maxillofacial prosthetics are a better option than conventional surgery when multiple procedures would be required. Also, surgical reconstruction may be limited by insufficient residual tissue, vascular compromise after radiation, age, the inadequacy of the donor site, or patient preference. Rehabilitation with maxillofacial prosthesis aims to restore an effective division between oral, nasal, and orbital cavities and gives faster reconstructive possibilities simplifying the post-surgery period and recovering an adequate patient lifestyle. Maxillofacial prosthetics are a subspecialty of prosthodontics which is a collaboration of ear, nose, and throat specialists, plastic surgeons, oral surgeons, and radiation oncologists in the case of cancer patients. Thus, it is a multidisciplinary branch which focuses on improving quality of life by preserving residual structures, restoring oral functions, and improving esthetic appearances [38].

The need for maxillofacial prostheses is increasing in recent years with the 6% increased prevalence of oral cancer, with the incidence being more in males in the ratio of 2:1 [39]. Maxillofacial defects can be classified as either intraoral or extra-oral. Intraoral include defects of the maxilla, mandible, tongue, soft palate, or hard palate and comprise mostly of birth defects like cleft lips. Extraoral defects include any other part of the head and neck. This defect inclines more towards trauma and tumor resurrection [39]. The obturators are prosthesis used to close palatal defects after maxillectomy, to restore masticatory function and to improve speech. Types of obturator can be broadly divided into surgical palatal obturator or fixed prosthetics, interim palatal obturator, and definitive palatal obturator. Surgical palatal obturator enables the palate and the pharyngeal muscles to contract, thereby restoring oral activities. The interim obturator is a removable prosthesis but is less preferable due to difficult retention techniques. Definitive palatal obturator extends into the nasal cavity instead of the hypopharynx and is prescribed for irreparable damage to the hard tissue or soft palate. Choosing the correct type of prostheses depends on the type of defect, age, location, and volume of residual tissue [40].

8. Conclusion

Throughout history, prosthetics have consistently improved on the degree of functional restoration possible for amputees and those with lost function. This improvement in their ability to perform ADL has led to improvements in quality of life. Recent trends in technology such as microprocessors, robotics, manufacturing, and biomechanics promise to improve both the functional and esthetic aspects of prosthetics, giving them a lifelike quality in both form and function. In this book, we explore some of these cutting-edge developments and how they will lead to better devices, ranging from limb replacements to retinal and maxillofacial prostheses. Future progress will be determined largely by patient needs, with economic restrictions leading to a desire for lower-cost yet reliable devices. Technological developments in neighboring fields such as aerospace and computer technology can lead to further innovative designs, making the future of prosthetics a promising one.

Author details

Shanthini Madhanagopal, Martin Burns, Dingyi Pei, Rohan Mukundhan, Helen Meyerson and Ramana Vinjamuri*
Sensorimotor Control Laboratory, Department of Biomedical Engineering, Stevens Institute of Technology, Hoboken, New Jersey, United States

*Address all correspondence to: ramana.vinjamuri@stevens.edu

References

[1] John C. Three Years of Work for Handicapped Men - A Report of the Activities of the Institute for Crippled and Disabled Men. New York; The Institute; 1920. pp. 19-24

[2] Marks LJ, Michael JW. Clinical review artificial limbs. BMJ. 2001;**323**:732-735

[3] Finch J. The art of medicine: The ancient origins of prosthetic medicine. Lancet. 2011;**377**(9765):548-549

[4] Kirkup J. A History of Limb Amputation. Weston Hill, Bath, UK: Springer; 2007. pp. 1-13

[5] Thurston AJ. The early history of artificial limbs. ANZ Journal of Surgery. 2007;**77**(12):1114-1119

[6] Norton KM. A Brief History of Prosthetics. InMotion. 2007;**17**(7):11-13

[7] Stryła W, Pogorzała AM, Kasior I, Nowakowski A. Limb amputations from the ancient times to the present. Polish Orthopaedics and Traumatology. 2013;**78**:155-166

[8] Fliegel O, Feuer SG. Historical development of lower-extremity prostheses. Orthopedic Prosthetic Appliance Journal. 1966;**47**(5):313-324

[9] Laferrier JZ, Gailey R. Advances in lower - limb prosthetic technology. Physical Medicine and Rehabilitation Clinics of North America. 2010;**21**:87-110

[10] Sheehan TP. Impact of limb loss in the United States. Physical Medicine & Rehabilitation Clinics of North America. 2014;**25**:9-28

[11] Webster JB, Hakimi KN, Williams RM, Turner AP, Norvell DC, Czerniecki JM. Prosthetic fitting, use, and satisfaction following lower-limb amputation: A prospective study. Journal of Rehabilitation Research and Development. 2012;**49**(10):1493-1504

[12] Ma VY, Chan L, The CKJ. Incidence, prevalence, costs and impact on disability of common conditions requiring rehabilitation in the US: Stroke, spinal cord injury, traumatic brain injury, multiple sclerosis, osteoarthritis, rheumatoid arthritis, limb loss, and back pain. Archives of Physical Medicine and Rehabilitation. 2014;**95**(5):986-995

[13] Lum PS, Godfrey SB, Brokaw EB, Holley RJ, Nichols D. Robotic approaches for rehabilitation of hand function after stroke. American Journal of Physical Medicine & Rehabilitation. 2012;**91**(11 Suppl 3): 242-251

[14] Mirelman A, Bonato P, Deutsch JE. Effects of training with a robot-virtual reality system compared with a robot alone on the gait of individuals after stroke. Stroke. 2009;**40**(1):169-174

[15] Resnik L, Etter K, Klinger SL, Kambe C. Using virtual reality environment to facilitate training with advanced upper-limb prosthesis. Journal of Rehabilitation Research and Development. 2011;**48**(6):707-718

[16] Lécuyer A, Lotte F, Reilly RB, Leeb R, Hirose M, Slater M. Brain-computer interfaces, virtual reality, and videogames. Computer (Long Beach Calif). 2008;**41**(10):66-72

[17] Shin JH, Ryu H, Jang SH. A task-specific interactive game-based virtual reality rehabilitation system for patients with stroke: A usability test and two clinical experiments. Journal of Neuroengineering and Rehabilitation. 2014;**11**(1):1-10

[18] Cameirao MS, Bermudez i Badia S, Duarte Oller E, Verschure PF. Neurorehabilitation using the virtual reality based rehabilitation gaming system: Methodology, design, psychometrics, usability and validation. Journal of Neuroengineering and Rehabilitation. 2010;**7**(1):48. Available from: http://jneuroengrehab.biomedcentral.com/articles/10.1186/1743-0003-7-48

[19] Wright TW, Hagen AD, Wood MB. Prosthetic usage in major upper extremity amputations. The Journal of Hand Surgery. 1995;**20A**(113):619-622

[20] Resnik L, Meucci MR, Lieberman-klinger S. Advanced upper limb prosthetic devices : Implications for upper limb rehabilitation. Archives of Physical Medicine and Rehabilitation. 2012;**93**(4):710-717

[21] Burger H, Marinček Č. Upper limb prosthetic use in Slovenia. Prosthetics and Orthotics International. 1994;**18**(1):25-33

[22] Lake C, Dodson R. Progressive upper limb prosthetics. Physical Medicine and Rehabilitation Clinics of North America. 2006;**17**:49-72

[23] Ziegler-graham K, Mackenzie EJ, Ephraim PL, Travison TG, Brookmeyer R, et al. Estimating the prevalence of limb loss in the United States: 2005 to 2050. Archives of Physical Medicine and Rehabilitation. 2008;**89**:422-429

[24] Deerochannawong C, Home PD, Alberti KG. A survey of lower limb amputation in diabetic patients. Diabetic Medicine. 1992;**9**:942-946

[25] Windrich M, Grimmer M, Christ O, Rinderknecht S, Beckerle P. Active lower limb prosthetics: A systematic review of design issues and solutions. Biomedical Engineering Online. 2016;**15**(3):5-19

[26] Edelstein EJE, Moroz A. Lower-limb prosthetics and orthotics : Clinical concepts. Journal of Sports Science and Medicine. 2011;**235**:2011

[27] Yang Q, Tong X, Schieb L, Vaughan A, Gillespie C, Wiltz JL. Vital signs: Recent trends in stroke death rates — United States, 2000 – 2015. Morbidity and Mortality Weekly Report Case Study. 2017;**66**(35):933-939

[28] Andersen RA, Burdick JW, Musallam S, Pesaran B, Cham JG. Cognitive neural prosthetics. Trends in Cognitive Sciences. 2004;**8**(11):486-493

[29] Terry Hambrecht F. Neural prostheses. Annual Review of Biophysics and Bioengineering. 1979;**1979**(8239-8267):239-269

[30] Santhanam G, Ryu SI, Yu BM, Afshar A, Shenoy KV. A high-performance brain-computer interface. International Journal of Natural Sciences. 2006;**442**(7099):195-198

[31] Greenberg RJ. Visual prostheses: A review. International Neuromodulation Society. 2000;**3**:161-165

[32] Palczewski K. Chemistry and biology of vision. The Journal of Biological Chemistry. 2012;**287**(3):1612-1619

[33] Chader GJ, Weiland J, Humayun MS. Artificial vision: Needs, functioning, and testing of a retinal electronic prosthesis. Progress in Brain Research. 2009;**175**:317-332

[34] Cohen E. Retinal prostheses. Kolb H, Fernandex E, Nelson R, editors. Webvision- The organisation of the Retina and Sisual System. Salt Lake City: University of Utah Health Sciences Center; 2018. pp. 1607-1629

[35] Wentai Liu MSH. Retinal Prosthesis. In: Biomicrosystems-IEEE International Solid-State Circuits Conference; 2004. pp. 1-2

[36] Gekeler F, Szurman P, Grisanti S, Weiler U, Claus R, Greiner T-O, et al. Compound subretinal prostheses with extra-ocular parts designed for human trials: successful long-term implantation in pigs. Graefe's Archive for Clinical and Experimental Ophthalmology. 2007;**245**(2):230-241

[37] Humayun MS, Dorn JD, Ahuja AK, Caspi A, Filley E, Salzmann J, et al. Preliminary 6 month results from the argus TM II epiretinal prosthesis feasibility study. In: International Conference of the IEEE Engineering in Medicine and Biology Society (EMBC); 2009. pp. 4566-4568

[38] Ralph S, Lloyd DDS, Bethesda M. Maxillofacial prosthesis. The Journal of the American Dental Association. 1944;**31**:1328-1335

[39] Gastaldi G, Palumbo L, Moreschi C, Gherlone EF, Capparé P. Prosthetic management of patients with Oro - Maxillo - facial defects: A long-term follow-up retrospective. ORAL & Implantology - Anno X. 2017;**3**(7):276-282

[40] Cardelli P, Bigelli E, Vertucci V, Balestra F, Montani M, Decarli S. Palatal obturators in patients after maxillectomy a case study. Oral & Implantology - Anno VII. 2014:86-92

Chapter 2

Estimation of Targeted-Reaching-Positions by Around-Shoulder Muscle Activities and Images from an Action Camera for Trans-Humeral Prosthesis Control

Yohei Muraguchi and Wenwei Yu

Abstract

For trans-humeral amputation, daily living tasks requiring bimanual coordination, such as lifting up a box, are most difficult, hence most urgent for a trans-humeral prosthesis to fulfill. However, in studies reported on trans-humeral prosthetic control, the states of the target objects, such as their size, relative pose and position, which are important for any real reaching and manipulation tasks, have not been taken into account. In our previous study, for a box lifting-up task, we investigated the possibility of using around-shoulder EMG (electromyogram), for identifying target-reaching-positions for the boxes with different configurations (relative pose and position). However, with only the around-shoulder EMG, it is impossible for the system to guide the prosthesis to hold or grasp target objects precisely and fast sufficiently. The purpose of this study is to explore the possibility of using both the image information from an action camera and around-shoulder EMG, to identify targeted-reaching-positions for various box configurations more accurately and more rapidly. Multinomial logistic regression was employed to realize both information integration of, and the target-reaching-position identification. A set of experiments were conducted. As a result, an average classification rate of 75.1% could be achieved for various box configurations.

Keywords: trans-humeral prosthesis, bimanual coordination, reaching motion, target objects information, logistic regression

1. Introduction

Fore-arm prostheses [1, 2] controlled by users' bio-signals have been the focus so far, while only fewer studies have been reported on prostheses for higher level amputees [3], due to the fact that there are fewer residual upper limb functions but higher DoFs (degree-of-freedoms) have to be controlled.

To solve this problem, several different approaches have been proposed. The iEEG (intracranial electroencephalogram), obtained from the intracranial electrodes embedded in the brain was used to control trans-humeral prostheses [4]. In [5], Kuiken et al. reported their research efforts to control trans-humeral prostheses using EMG by TMR (targeted muscle reinnervation) technology. By the above-mentioned methods, an intuitive user-prosthesis interface could be achieved using the bio-signals with more direct information of intended motions, however, the problems are clear: they are invasive and need surgery, which costs high, and may cause physical and mental burden to patients.

In [6, 7], the EMG (electromyogram) signals from the around-shoulder area (ASA), and in [8], the EMG from the ASA, together with additional motion-related EEG were used, and machine learning methods were employed to explore the limited information.

Bimanual coordination between one's healthy arm and its prosthetic counterpart, in bimanual tasks such as holding a bottle with one hand while opening its lid with another hand, operating a car handle, and lifting up a box, was proposed as one solution [9–15]. This is because at first, the needs of trans-humeral prostheses might mostly come from the bimanual coordination, since in daily living, there are many tasks that need the coordination of the limbs of both sides [16], while most amputees can use their healthy (normal) side to complete most tasks that do not need bimanual coordination. Secondly, more information for controlling trans-humeral prostheses can be acquired from both coordinating sides, since the required behavior of the prostheses could be estimated from not only the residual stumps, but also the motion and motor behavior of the normal side, too.

However, in the studies of bimanual coordination mentioned before, the states of target objects, such as their relative position, size, and pose, which are important for any real manipulation and reaching tasks, has not been taken into consideration. In a typical bimanual coordination task: lifting up a box by two hands, the target-reaching-position for a trans-humeral prosthesis to reach varies depending on the state of the box. For this reason, it is necessary to take into consideration the states of target objects when identifying the target-reaching-position of the healthy arm for realizing the bimanual coordination for the users of trans-humeral prostheses.

Similarly, bimanual coordination has been addressed in robotics [17]. In a study on bimanual box grasping by a humanoid robot, the concept of grasping stability was used to deal with the different states of the box [18].

In our previous study, we explored the possibility of identifying target-reaching-positions with respect to various box configurations (box size and relative pose) and investigated the features highly generalized for unknown data: i.e., those that could enable the classifiers to be trained by fewer box configurations. However, it was made clear that, with only the ASA EMG, it is impossible for the system to guide the prosthesis to hold or grasp target objects precisely and fast sufficiently for the daily living activities.

This study has two relevant purposes, throughout the experiments and analyses for the bimanual box lifting task. The first is to explore the possibility of identifying the target-reaching-positions with respect to various box configurations, using two signal sources: bio-signals detected from the around-shoulder area and images from an action camera. Here a box configuration specifies the pose and the position of a box relative to the user. The reason for using the bio-signal only from around-shoulder area is that the sensors at the distal sites are more likely to be affected by external perturbation, moreover, around shoulder sensors configuration could be also applied to the amputated side. On the other hand, the reason for attaching the camera near the shoulder is that the camera there does not limit the use of both arms in practical use even in a wearable setting, and its positional relation with the trans-humeral prosthesis is straightforward. Classifiers are trained to identify the intended target-reaching-positions for different box configurations.

The second is to explore the optimal way to integrate the information from the two signal sources, to realize fast and accurate target-reaching-position. Since only with the fast and accurate estimation, there could be sufficient time for controlling the trans-humeral prosthesis to match the healthy upper limb.

2. Feature selection and classification for target-reaching-positions

2.1 Feature selection

Three hundred and ninety eight features (i.e., 8 EMG sensors × 10-time steps + 28 ratio of WL × 10-time steps + 8 total sums of WL + 28 ratio of total sum of WL + box pose + box position) were calculated from the measured data. Apparently, using all the features for classification may cause training problems, such as flattening or over-fitting. In this study, the Akaike information criterion (AIC) [19] was used for feature selection.

$$AIC = 2k - 2\,ln(L) \tag{1}$$

Here, k is the number of parameters in the statistical model, and L is the maximized value of the likelihood function for it.

Method of incrementally increasing and decreasing representative variables in [20] was used to select features. That is, if the AIC does not decrease when the next feature is added, the feature selection ends. To decide the initial values for the selection, the ratio between interclass variance and in-class variance in [21] was used. The feature with the largest ratio is adopted as the initial value.

2.2 Evaluation of the features and classification of the target-reaching-positions in the multinomial logistic regression

Multinomial logistic regression analysis was employed as the classifier. The method is called a multinomial logit model, which is one of several natural extensions of the binary logit origin. This multinomial logit model counts the relative probability of being in one category versus being in a reference category, k, using a linear combination of predictor variables. Consequently, the probability of each outcome is expressed as a nonlinear function of p predictor variables [22].

The multinomial logit model can be expressed as the following equations:

$$ln\left(\frac{\pi_1}{\pi_k}\right) = \alpha_1 + \beta_{11}X_1 + \beta_{12}X_2 + \cdots + \beta_{1p}X_p,$$

$$ln\left(\frac{\pi_2}{\pi_k}\right) = \alpha_2 + \beta_{21}X_1 + \beta_{22}X_2 + \cdots + \beta_{2p}X_p,$$

$$\vdots$$

$$\ln\left(\frac{\pi_{k-1}}{\pi_k}\right) = \alpha_{(k-1)} + \beta_{(k-1)1}X_1 + \beta_{(k-1)2}X_2 + \cdots + \beta_{(k-1)p} \tag{2}$$

where $\pi_j = P\,(y = j)\,(j = 1, 2, \ldots, k)$ is the probability of an outcome being in category j, k is the number of response categories, $\pi_j = P\,(y = j)$, and p is the number of predictor variables. A total of j-1 equations was solved simultaneously to estimate the coefficients. The coefficients in the model express the effects of the predictor variables on the relative risk or the log odds of being in category j versus the reference category, here k, [22]. When used in classification, the probability of each label can be obtained from the above equations and the feature obtained by measurement. The label with the highest probability is the classification result.

In the feature selection by AIC, a feature is selected by its compatibility with the previously selected features. Therefore, in essence, the features selected earlier are not guaranteed to the best. On the other hand, coefficient, and the p value of the coefficient of the feature by the logistic regression (coefficient, p value of the coefficient) can represent how the feature affects the classification. The feature with the smallest p value affects the classification the most. The reason for using AIC as feature selection is that the logistic regression equation could not deal with directly a large number of predictor variables, i.e., features. For the above reasons, we performed the feature selection using AIC, and feature evaluation logistic regression.

Regarding classification methods, SVM [23] and neural networks [1, 2] are well used for bio-signals. However, in this research, not only the classification but also the information integration based on feature selection and evaluation is required, which is difficult for both SVM and neural networks. Contrarily, the multinomial logistic regression can perform a dual role of classification and feature evaluation. In addition, since classification results of the multinomial logistic regression come with the probability, it is also possible to evaluate the ambiguity of the classification. Furthermore, the multinomial logistic regression uses only j-1 (j: number of categories) weighted sum for classification, its computational cost shall be lower than that of SVM and neural networks.

The difficulty of this research lies in the fact that, the reaching motion to the same relative position of the box with different box configuration (relative pose and position) should be classified as the same class, and in some cases, as the box position changes, even though the actual target-reaching-position is almost the same, the label of the target-reaching-position that should be classified shall be completely different. For example, the back of one box placed at a certain position, and the front of another box placed at a displacement of the box width are the planes with same position. If with only EMG, the reaching motion to both planes would be identified as the same, though they should be classified as the different ones. Therefore, it is necessary to introduce in some forms the box configuration information, and investigate how to integrate the two types of signals.

We compared between two datasets. Dataset 1 used EMG only; dataset used EMG and the box configuration (relative pose and position). Also, the classification was performed in two steps. In step 1, the upper side of the box (RP1, 2, 3) and the bottom side of the box (RP4, 5, 6) were classified. In step 2, in the case where it was classified as the upper side of the box in step 1, classification of RP1, RP2, RP3 was performed. If it was classified as the bottom side of the box, RP4, RP5, RP6 were classified. When the classification result is correct in both steps, the classification rate was increased. In that case, the classification rate was calculated by leave-one-out cross validation.

Feature extraction and feature selection were performed every 0.1 s from the start of motions. Feature selection was performed for each subject and classifier (for the upper side of the box and the bottom side of the box, for RP1, RP2 and RP3, for RP4, RP5 and RP6), and the feature was not unified among subjects. After that, the multinomial logistic regression was constructed using the selected features from the data until a specified elapsed time step, and the change of classification rate was investigated each dataset.

3. Measurement experiment

3.1 Subjects

Three male healthy subjects, of age 23, with no known history of neurological abnormalities or musculo-skeletal disorders, participated in the experiments. They were informed about the experimental procedures and asked to provide a signed consent.

3.2 Experiment procedure

The subjects were required to stand comfortably in front of a table. Before starting a new trial, they were asked to rest the palm of their dominant hand naturally open. They were instructed to move their dominant hand towards one of the six target-reaching-positions on the side of a box, for the purpose of lifting it up (**Figure 1**), after pushing a button to denote a new trial.

The size of the box used during the experiment was 260 × 310 × 165 mm (Length × Width × Height). The box was placed in one of four different poses, and three different positions relative to the subject, as denoted in **Figures 2** and **3**, respectively. The subjects were asked to reach a total of five times for each box configuration, giving a total of 360 (6 positions × 4 poses of box × 3 position of box × 5 times) trials. The subjects were required to do the reaching motion with 1.0 s, following the tempo of a metronome. They could rest for a few seconds between each trial. Muscle activity, skin surface undulation during the motions were recorded with the sensors and devices described in the next subsection.

3.3 Devices

In the experiment, eight EMG sensors (Trigno, DELSYS), were used to measure the muscle activity. The sensor signals were recorded using Powelab 16/35 (AD instruments), at a sampling frequency of 400 Hz. Generally, the sampling frequency used for muscle activity recording is 1 kHz or more, but because no frequency-domain features are to be used in the classification, as shown in the next subsection, the sampling frequency was decreased.

The eight EMG sensors were placed on the skin surface of eight different muscles around the shoulder: Latissimus dorsi, Deltoid middle strand, Deltoid front strand, Deltoid rear strand, Triceps branchii, Middle part of trapezius, Descending part of trapezius, Pectoralis major, as shown in **Figure 4**, were selected according to the shoulder anatomy [24].

The action camera was attached to the shoulder mouth. Then, the image during the reaching motion measurement was acquired. However, this study no information was acquired using image processing. Although the action camera and the algorithms to process the images have been determined, in this study, because it is the integration of information from different signal sources that is to be investigated, the information of relative pose and position the of box was directly used.

3.4 Feature extraction

The EMG signals were processed by a 1 Hz high-pass filter.

The features were based on the waveform length (WL) of filtered raw signals. WL is a measure of complexity of the EMG signal, which is defined as the

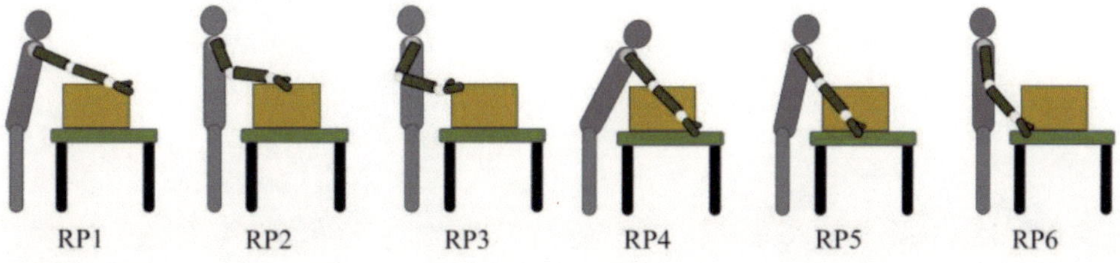

Figure 1.
Reaching position (RP: reaching position).

cumulative length of the waveform over the time segment [25]. The following features calculated.

1. WL in the segmentation delimited by every time step (0.1 s) and the ratio of WL of each two EMG channels in that interval

2. The total sum of WL until a specified elapsed time and Ratio of WL of each two channels in that interval

Regarding the relative pose and position information of the box, the angle of the reaching side (as shown in **Figure 2**), and the distance between the subject and the box (as shown in **Figure 3**) were used, respectively. To simulate the error possibly caused by image processing, and investigate the tolerance of the classification to configuration deviation, a simulated error was added to the configuration information.

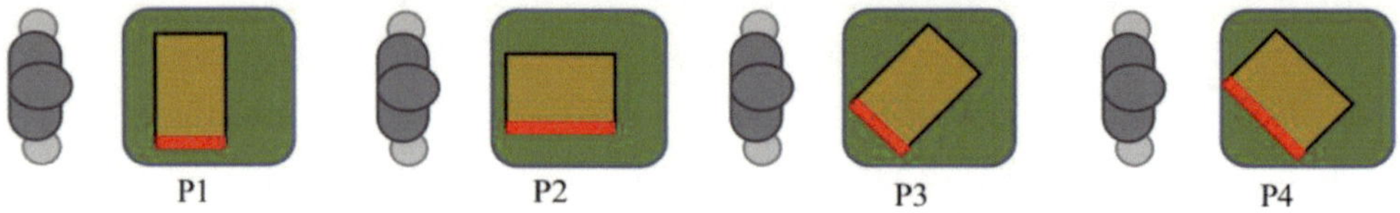

Figure 2.
Box pose (P: pose).

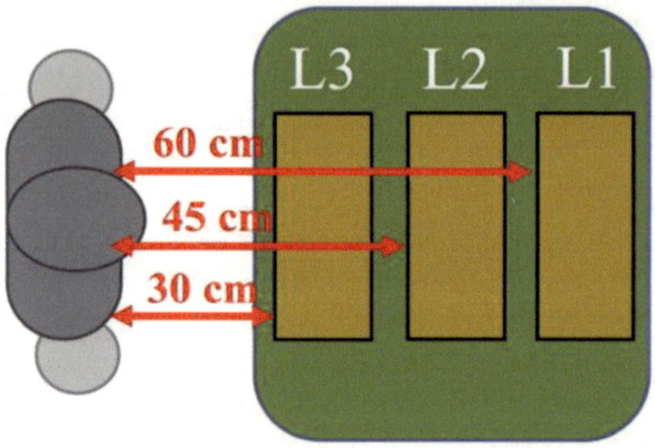

Figure 3.
Box position (L: position).

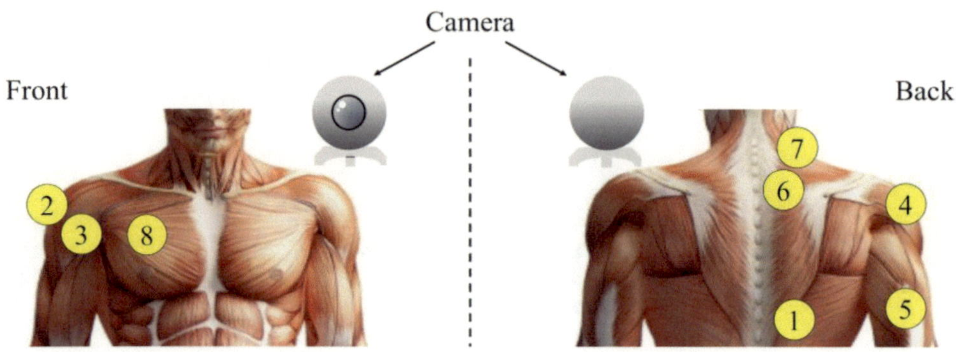

Figure 4.
The position of the sensors.

In the analysis for classification rate (Sections 4.1 and 4.2), evaluation of features (Section 4.3), random values (−0.5 to +0.5) created using MATLAB were added to the box pose and box position. Here, 0.5 mean 50% of the angular interval between different poses (45° × 0.5 = 22.5°) (see **Figure 2**), or distance interval between different relative positions (15 cm/2 = 7.5 cm) (see **Figure 3**). In the analysis of the effect of simulated error (Section 4.4), four levels of simulated errors: 0, ±0.5, ±0.75, ±1.0 were added. That is, the maximal actual distance (position) error is ±15 cm (±1.0) and, the maximal actual angle (pose) error is ±45° (±1.0). That is, the maximum error given is same as the angular interval between box poses.

The box pose and box position information were introduced as categorical variables. The box pose information P1 and P2 are set to 1, P3 and P4 are set to 2 in **Figure 2**. The box position information L1, L2 and L3, as shown in **Figure 3**, were set to 1, 2, and 3, respectively. Also, all features were standardized using the Z score for evaluation of selected features. For a random variable X with mean μ and standard deviation σ, the z-score of a value x is

$$z = \frac{(x - \mu)}{\delta} \quad (3)$$

4. Results and discussion

4.1 Comparison using classification rates

Figures 5–7 show the classification rate at each elapsed time step of the reaching motion for each subject. RPi (i = 1–6) in each figure represents a reaching positions, the meaning of the digit i can be found in **Figure 1**. At the end of the reaching motion, the classification rate achieved by classification with only EMG and that of EMG + box configuration information was 60.0 and 75.1%, on average for all subjects, respectively. It is clear that the classification rate was greatly improved by integrating the box configuration information and ASA muscle activities.

In **Figures 5–7**, the legend markers RP 123, RP 456, RP upper_and_bottom represent the result of classifying relative position 1, 2, 3, relative position 4, 5, 6, and relative position upper row and bottom row, respectively.

As seen from **Figures 5(a), 6(a)**, and **7(a)**, when using only EMG as the features, at the elapsed time step of 0.5 seconds, the classification rate of RP 123, RP 456 and RP upper and bottom was 55.4, 59.6, and 84.3% on average for all subjects, respectively. At the end of the reaching motion, the classification rate of RP 123, RP 456 and RP upper and bottom was 68.9, 62.2 and 91.5% on average for all subjects, respectively.

In contrast, when using the EMG and the box configuration (relative pose and position) information as the features, at the elapsed time step of 0.5 s, the classification rate of RP 123, RP 456 and RP upper and bottom was 76.9, 74.4 and 84.5% on average for all subjects, respectively. At the end of the reaching motion was 83.5, 82.2 and 90.9% on average for all subjects, respectively.

It can be seen from these results that, no clear classification rate increase was observed even if the state of the box was introduced in classification of the box top and bottom. On the other hand, it is found that the box configuration is effective for identifying the depth of the reaching motion, since an increase of about 20% was observed.

Although the classification rates are not as high as those in the studies for recognizing the motions of hands and fingers [1, 2, 4], considering the disadvantages brought by the boxes with different configurations, and limited EMG measurement sites, the results are acceptable. Moreover, the results are comparable to those in the research on complex motions [26, 27], in which the classification rate reported was around 70% too. So in the following analysis, 70% is used as the threshold for investigating the real-time characteristics.

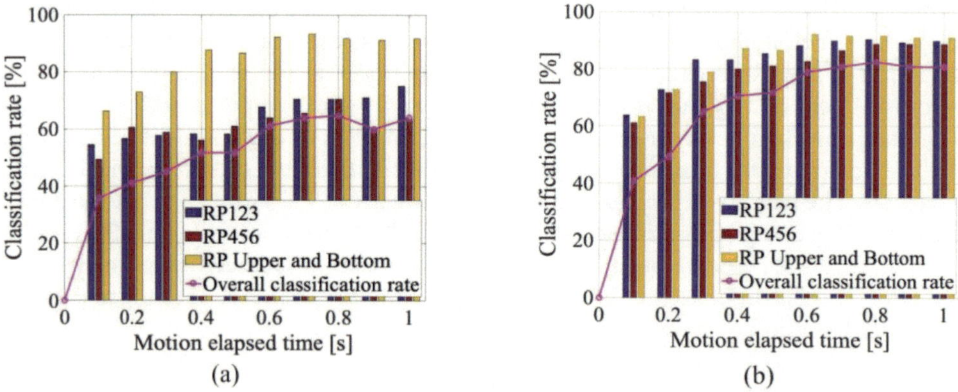

Figure 5.
*Classification rate at each elapsed time step of reaching motion (subject A, (a) uses only EMG for the feature, (b) uses EMG and box configurations (pose, position) for the feature, RP: reaching position, see **Figure 1**).*

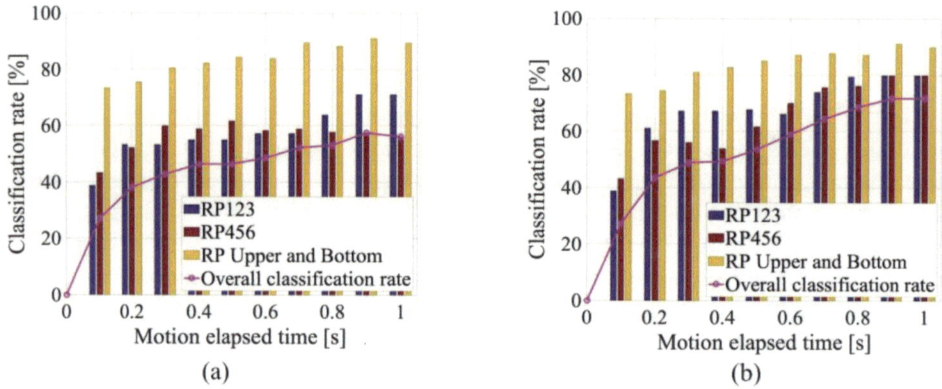

Figure 6.
*Classification rate at each elapsed time step of reaching motion (subject B, (a) uses only EMG for the feature, (b) uses EMG and box configurations (pose, position) for the feature, RP: reaching position, see **Figure 1**).*

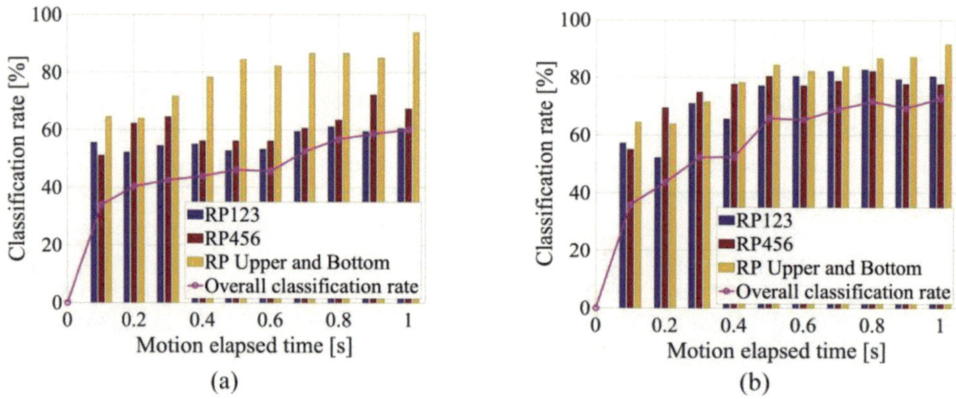

Figure 7.
*Classification rate at each elapsed time step of reaching motion (subject C, (a) uses only EMG for the feature, (b) uses EMG and box configurations (pose, position) for the feature, RP: reaching position, see **Figure 1**).*

Table 1 shows the timing when the classification rate exceeded 70%, and the classification rate at 0.5 seconds for each subject. As seen from the table, when using only EMG as the features, the classification rate did not exceed 70% for any subjects. When using the EMG and box configuration as the features, subject A, B, C achieved 70% at the timing of 0.4 0.9 and 0.8 s, respectively. Also, when using only EMG as the features, the classification rate at 0.5 seconds was 51.7, 46.4, and 46.1%, for subject A, B, and C, respectively. In contrast, when using the EMG and box configuration as the features, subject A, B and C achieved 71.7, 53.6, and 65.8%, respectively. By introducing the box configuration information as the features, the classification rate of subject A, B, and C increased by 20.2, 7.2, and 19.7%, respectively. From these results, it is clear that, the information of box configuration enables more accurate and faster classification.

4.2 Comparison using classification probabilities

Figure 8 shows the probabilities obtained by the logistic regression at the end of the reaching motion of the subject A. In the figure, (a) shows the case using only EMG as the features, (b) shows the case using both EMG and box configuration (pose, position) information as the features. A reaching position with the highest resultant probability was counted as the classification result.

From **Figure 8(1, 2)**, it can be seen that in the classification of box upper and bottom, high probabilities were achieved even when only EMG was used as the features. From **Figure 8(3–8)**, when only the EMG was used as the features, the probabilities were low even if the classification results were correct (a), but when both EMG and box configuration were used, the probabilities showed a clear difference for classification, which means that ambiguity decreases by introducing the box configuration information as features.

4.3 Evaluation of selected features

Tables 2 and **3** show the features selected using AIC, the coefficients of each feature in the logistic regression, p value in the classification of upper and bottom side reaching position. **Table 3** have the similar layout, showing the features selected using AIC, coefficients of each feature in the logistic regression, and p value for classification of RP1/2/3, and RP4/5/6, respectively. In **Tables 2** and **3**, the selected features were arranged in the selected order.

From **Table 2**, it is clear that, for the classification of RP upper and bottom side, the box configuration information (both the pose and position), was not selected by the AIC selection process. As can be seen from **Table 3**, for the classification of RP1/2/3 and RP4/5/6, the box pose and position were selected. Moreover, the p value of the box position is the smallest, which means the box position is the most contributing feature for the classification.

	The timing exceeding the classification rate of 70% [s]		The classification rate at 0.5 s [%]	
Subject	Only EMG	EMG and box configuration	Only EMG	EMG and box configuration
A	Not exceeded	0.4	51.7	71.7
B	Not exceeded	0.8	46.4	53.6
C	Not exceeded	0.9	46.1	65.8

Table 1.
The timing exceeding the classification rate of 70% and the classification rate at 0.5 s each dataset.

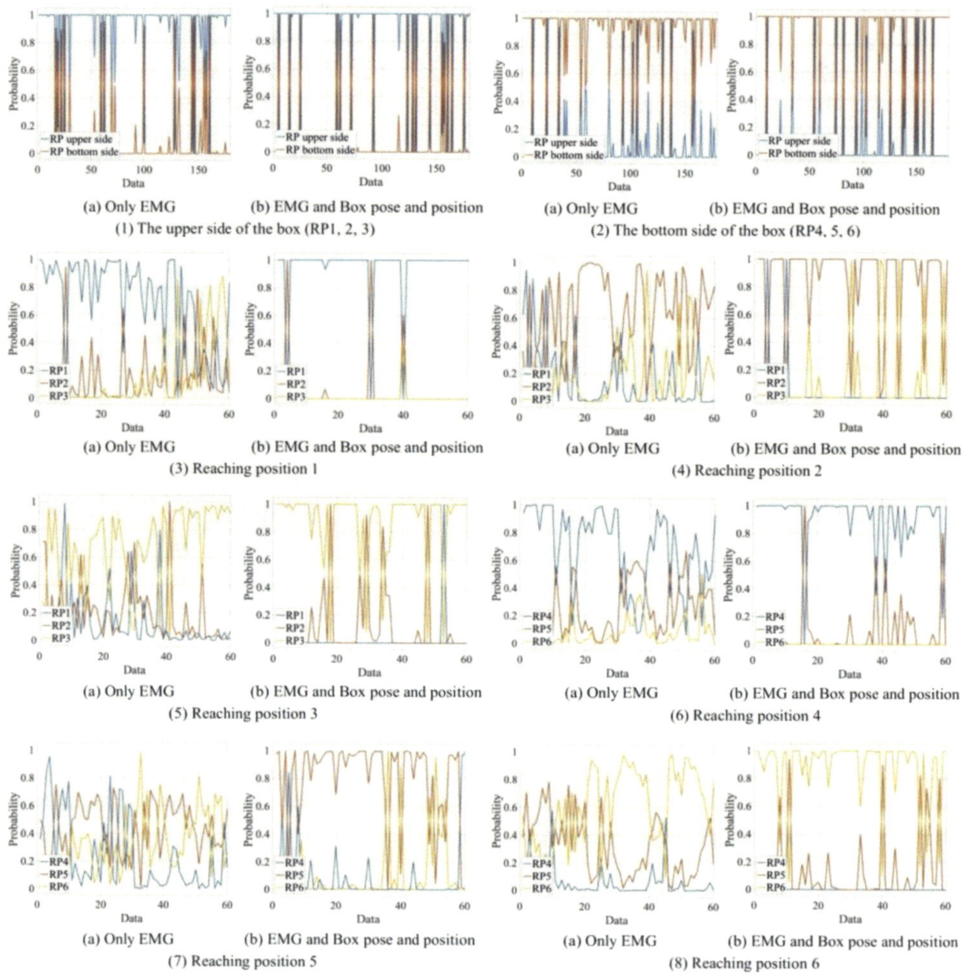

Figure 8.
The probability obtained by the logistic regression equation (subject A, at the end of the reaching motion, (a) uses only EMG for the feature, (b) uses EMG and box configurations (pose, position) for the feature, the reaching position with the highest probability is the identification result).

4.4 Influence of the simulated errors for box configuration information

If the box configuration information is calculated from the image processing from the action camera, errors occur due to the influence of noise, measurement error and the other system errors. Therefore, in this research, the tolerable range of the error was investigated by adding simulated error to the true box configuration.

Figure 9 shows the influence of the simulated error level of the box configuration information on the classification rate of each subject. As seen from the figure, the classification rate decreased when the error level was increased in all subjects. In the case of subject A, even if the highest level error, 1.0 was given, a classification rate exceeding 70% was obtained. In the case of subject B, when the simulated error level 0.75 or more was given, the classification rate was lower than 70%. For subject C, when simulated error level 1.0 was given, the classification rate fell below 70%. From these results, it can be said that the error level should be controlled to 0.5 or less (position: 7.5 cm or less, posture: 22.5° or less).

Selected feature	Coefficient	p value	Selected feature	Coefficient	p value
Intercept	0.03	0.874	34, rdWL	1.76	3.85E-5
137, vdWL	1.23	0.001	127, vdWL	1.55	0.003
89, rdWL	−0.88	0.024	93, rdWL	−2.91	1.23E-7
99, rdWL	2.21	1.90E-8	53, rdWL	−0.84	0.004
152, rtWL	1.15	0.001	87, rdWL	1.12	0.001
117, vdWL	1.38	9.48E-6	180, vtWL	1.78	4.16E-4
84, rdWL	1.10	0.001	176, vtWL	−1.26	2.69E-4
32, rdWL	−1.55	5.64E-7	21, rdWL	0.89	0.006
65, rdWL	−1.58	6.11E-5	61, rdWL	0.70	0.002
85, rdWL	−2.11	2.70E-6	111, rdWL	0.99	0.18
102, rdWL	−1.80	1.79E-4			

The meaning of the symbols: r, the ratio of WL; the value of WL; t, total sum for the whole period of the reaching motion; d, segmentation delimited by every time step (0.1 s). The ID number and type of features are expressed as follows. rdWL(1–112): the ratio of WL in the segmentation delimited by every time step (0.1 s); vdWL(113–144): WL in the segmentation delimited by every time step (0.1 s); rtWL(145–172): the ratio of the total sum of WL until a specified elapsed time; vtWL(173–180): the total sum of WL until a specified elapsed time; BP(181): the box pose and BL(182): the box position; p value represents statistical significance of coefficient.

Table 2.
In classification of RP upper and bottom side, feature selected using AIC, coefficients of the logistic regression equation, p value (dataset: EMG and box configuration).

Selected feature	Coefficient	p value	Coefficient	p value
	π4 versus π6		**π5 versus π6**	
(a) In classification of RP1/2/3				
Intercept	−2.69	0.011	3.29	1.05E-6
154, rtWL	10.94	2.30E-10	2.24	0.046
182, BL	14.50	3.34E-17	6.20	6.49E-8
175, vtWL	7.94	0.002	4.78	0.017
181, BP	7.50	1.67E-14	2.74	2.02E-6
177, vtWL	7.72	2.69E-8	2.29	0.017
169, rtWL	−1.69	0.005	−1.12	0.006
115, vdWL	−6.98	8.06E-6	−1.07	0.287
152, rtWL	−14.31	4.23E-10	−2.48	2.81E-4
	π4 versus π6		**π5 versus π6**	
(b) In classification of RP4/5/6				
Intercept	1.65	0.134	3.56	4.61E-4
145, vdWL	−2.89	0.009	−1.04	0.161
182, BL	8.17	1.98E-9	5.43	3.83E-6
131, vdWL	3.88	0.004	3.24	0.009
181, BP	5.17	1.33E-8	3.37	1.56E-5
174, vtWL	8.61	4.88E-5	5.82	0.003
8, rdWL	−3.36	8.58E-4	−2.21	0.007

Selected feature	Coefficient	p value	Coefficient	p value
	π4 versus π6		π5 versus π6	
17, rdWL	−2.15	0.087	−0.96	0.420

The meaning of the symbols: r, the ratio of WL; the value of WL; t, total sum for the whole period of the reaching motion; d, segmentation delimited by every time step (0.1 s). The ID number and type of features are expressed as follows. rdWL(1–112): the ratio of WL in the segmentation delimited by every time step (0.1 s); vdWL(113–144): WL in the segmentation delimited by every time step (0.1 s); rtWL(145–172): the ratio of the total sum of WL until a specified elapsed time; vtWL(173–180): the total sum of WL until a specified elapsed time; BP(181): the box pose and BL(182): the box position; p value represents statistical significance of coefficient.

Table 3.
Feature selected using AIC, coefficients of the logistic regression equation, p value (dataset: EMG and box configuration).

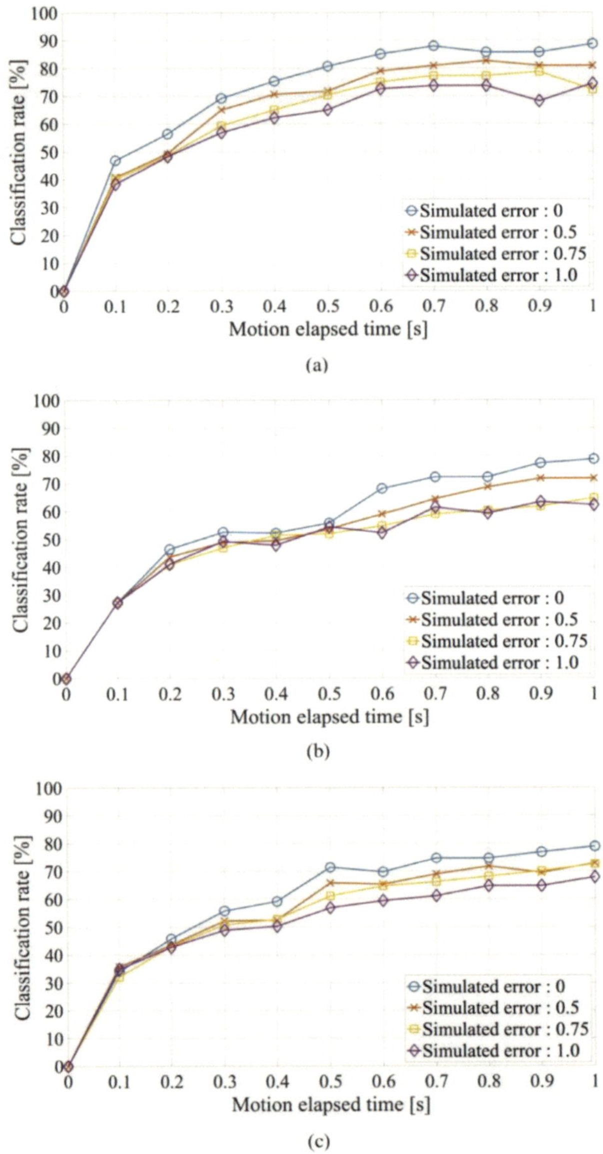

Figure 9.
Influence of box configuration information on classification rate due to error (±1.0: Corresponding to 15 cm for position, and 45° for pose). (a) Subject A, (b) subject B, and (c) subject C.

5. Conclusion

In this research, we employed multinomial logistic regression to realize both information integration of two signal sources: images and around-shoulder EMG, and the target-reaching-position identification for 12 box configuration (pose 4 × position 3).

A high classification rate was achieved using both information sources. It was found that the box configuration information contributes to the classification of the depth of the reaching motion. Moreover, since the timing at which the classification rate exceeds 70% greatly differs from each subject, it is considered that the optimal classification timing might be individual dependent. Furthermore, the classification rate decreased when the error level was increased in all subjects.

In the experiment, we only changed the box position in the depth direction relative to the subject. Lateral changes of the box position relative to the subject shall be investigated, in the near future. Moreover, the effect of the box configuration information calculated from the real images captured by the active camera should be studied and compared with the results of this study. Since the error caused by the image acquisition and processing, as well as the real computational cost shall affect the information integration. Finally, the system should be finally validated with the data from amputee subjects.

Acknowledgements

This work was supported by JSPS Grant-in-Aid for Scientific Research (B) 17H02129.

Author details

Yohei Muraguchi[1] and Wenwei Yu[2]*

1 Graduate School of Engineering, Chiba University, Chiba, Japan

2 Center for Frontier Medical Engineering, Chiba University, Chiba, Japan

*Address all correspondence to: yuwill@faculty.chiba-u.jp

References

[1] Nishikawa D, Yu W, Yokoi H, Kakazu Y. On-line learning method for EMG prosthetic hand controlling. Electronics and Communications in Japan. 2001;**84**(10):35-46

[2] Nishikawa D, Yu W, Yokoi H, Kakazu Y. On-line supervising mechanism for learning data in surface electromyogram motion classifiers. Systems and Computers in Japan. 2002;**33**(14):1-11

[3] DEKA Research & Development Corp. LUKE Arm Details [Online]. Available from: http://www.mobiusbionics.com/luke-arm/ [Accessed: December 4, 2018]

[4] Fifer MS et al. Simultaneous neural control of simple reaching and grasping with the modular prosthetic limb using intracranial EEG. IEEE Transactions on Neural Systems and Rehabilitation Engineering. 2014;**22**(3):695-705

[5] Kuiken TA et al. Targeted muscle reinnervation for real-time myoelectric control of multifunction artificial arms. JAMA: The Journal of the American Medical Association. 2009;**301**(6):619-628

[6] Horiuchi Y, Kishi T, Gonzalez J, Yu W. A study on classification of upper limb motions from around-shoulder muscle activities. In: 2009 IEEE International Conference on Rehabilitation Robotics (ICORR 2009); 2009. pp. 311-315

[7] Gonzalez J. Classification of upper limb motions from around-shoulder muscle activities: Hand biofeedback. The Open Medical Informatics Journal. 2010;**4**(2):74-80

[8] Jacobo FV, Yee CL, Kahori K, Yu W. 3D continuos hand motion reconstruction from dual EEG and EMG recordings. In: ICIIBMS 2015—International Conference on Intelligent Informatics and Biomedical Sciences; November 2016. pp. 101-108

[9] Mahira T, Imamogh N, Gomez-Tames J, Kita K, Yu W. Modeling bimanual coordination using back propagation neural network and radial basis function network. In: IEEE International Conference on Robotics and Biomimetics; 2014. pp. 1356-1361

[10] Uoi T, Inohira E, Yokoi H. Generation of movements used in daily life using a bimanual coordinated motion generation system for myoelectric upper limb prostheses. Transactions of Japanese Society for Medical and Biological Engineering. 2012;**50**:337-344

[11] Vasan G, Pilarski PM. Learning from demonstration: Teaching a myoelectric prosthesis with an intact limb via reinforcement learning. In: IEEE International Conference on Rehabilitation Robotics (ICORR); 2017. pp. 1457-1464

[12] Choi H et al. Improved prediction of bimanual movements by a two-staged (effector-then-trajectory) decoder with epidural ECoG in nonhuman primates. Journal of Neural Engineering. 2018;**15**(1):1-10. Article 016011

[13] Strazzulla I, Nowak M, Controzzi M, Cipriani C, Castellini C. Online bimanual manipulation using surface electromyography and incremental learning. IEEE Transactions on Neural Systems and Rehabilitation Engineering. 2017;**25**(3):227-234

[14] Toyokura M, Muro I, Komiya T, Obara M. Activation in the frontomesial cortex during bimanually coordinated movement: Analysis using functional magnetic resonance imaging. Rehabilitation Medicine: The Japanese

Journal of Rehabilitation Medicine, The Japanese association of rehabilitation medicine. 2000;**37**(10):662-668

[15] Tazoe T. The effectiveness of bimanual coordination in stroke hemiplegia. Uehara Memorial Life Science Foundation Study Reports. 2012;**26**:1-4

[16] Kamakura N. Shapes of Hands, Movements of Hands. Tokyo: Medical, Dental and Pharmacological Publication Co.; 1989

[17] Vahrenkamp N, Boge C, Welke K, Asfour T, Walterl J, Dillmann R. Visual servoing for dual arm motions on a humanoid robot. In: IEEE-RAS International Conference on Humanoid Robots; 2009. pp. 208-214

[18] Huebner K, Welke K, Przybylski M, Vahrenkamp N, Asfour T, Kragic D. Grasping known objects with humanoid robots: A box-based approach. In: IEEE International Conference on Advanced Robotics; 2009

[19] Akaike H. A new look at the statistical model identification. IEEE Transactions on Automatic Control. 1974;**19**(6):716-723

[20] Sato Y. Classification of Multivariate Data–Discriminan Analysis, Cluster Analysis. Tokyo: Asakura Publishing Co., Ltd.; 2009

[21] Han M, Liu X. Feature selection techniques with class separability for multivariate time series. Neurocomputing. 2013;**110**:29-34

[22] The MathWorks, Inc. Multinomial Models for Nominal Responses [Online]. Available from: https://jp.mathworks.com/help/stats/multinomial-models-for-nominal-responses.html?lang=en [Accessed: January 2019]

[23] Subasi A. Classification of EMG signals using PSO optimized SVM for diagnosis of neuromuscular disorders. Computers in Biology and Medicine. 2013;**43**(5):576-586

[24] Nakamura R, Saito H. Basic Kinesiology. 6th ed. Tokyo: Medical, Dental and Pharmacological Publication Co.; 2003

[25] Phinyomark A, Phukpattaranont P, Limsakul C. Feature reduction and selection for EMG signal classification. Expert Systems with Applications. 2012;**39**(8):7420-7431

[26] Itou T, Terao M, Nagata J, Yoshida M. Mouse cursor control system using electrooculogram signals. In: IEEE Engineering in Medicine and Biology Society; 2001. pp. 1368-1369

[27] Jung KK, Kim JW, Lee HK, Chung SB, Eom KH. EMG pattern classification using spectral estimation and neural network. In: Proceedings of the SICE Annual Conference; 2007. pp. 1108-1111

Chapter 3

Hybrid Neuroprosthesis for Lower Limbs

Percy Nohama, Guilherme Nunes Nogueira Neto
and Maira Ranciaro

Abstract

Assistive technologies have been proposed for the locomotion of people with spinal cord injury (SCI). One of them is the neuroprosthesis that arouses the interest of developers and health professionals bearing in mind the beneficial effects promoted in people with SCI. Thus, the first session of this chapter presents the principles of human motility and the impact that spinal cord injury causes on a person's mobility. The second session presents functional electrical stimulation as a solution for the immobility of paralyzed muscles. It explains the working principles of constituent modules and main stimulatory parameters. The third session introduces the concepts and characteristics of neural prosthesis hybridization. The last two sessions present and discuss examples of hybrid neuroprostheses. Such systems employ hybrid assistive lower limb strategies to evoke functional movements in people with SCI, associating the motor effects of active and/or passive orthoses to a functional electrical stimulation (FES) system. Examples of typical applications of FES in rehabilitation are discussed.

Keywords: spinal cord injury, locomotion, lower limb,
functional electrical stimulation, neuroprosthesis, hybrid neuroprosthesis

1. Introduction

1.1 Human motricity and the impact of spinal cord injury

There are three forms of human motricity: voluntary, involuntary, and reflex. Voluntary motricity is represented by the pyramidal system. Cortical motor cells and their extensions form the corticospinal pathway. The motor system is bineuronal and extends from the cerebral cortex to the myoneural junction. The first neuron (central motor neuron) has its cell body in the cerebral cortex from where its axon goes out. Synaptic endings occur in the anterior roots of the spinal cord, where they connect with the second neuron (peripheral motor neuron). This is the so-called pyramidal path. The axons of the pyramidal path pass through the oval center, the inner capsule, and arrive in the brainstem where most of their fibers cross the midline. These axons follow along with the lateral cord of the spinal cord and end up connecting the peripheral motor neuron in the anterior root of the spinal cord.

Involuntary motricity involves the extrapyramidal system. Cell bodies stem from the various nuclei of the base and are associated with areas of the motor cortex, pre-motor, and subthalamic nuclei. There are several paths such as rubrospinal, reticulospinal, vestibulospinal, and cephalospinal paths. The extrapyramidal system and its pathways harmonize the voluntary motor system, guarantee the automatic motricity, and control the postural reflexes of spinal and vestibulocerebellar origins.

Reflex motricity depends on the pyramidal and extrapyramidal systems and represents only a few spinal reflexes.

Peripheral motor neurons are part of the peripheral nervous system (PNS) and are organized into motor units. Nerve fibers protract from the anterior roots of the spinal cord to muscle fibers and organs of muscular proprioception called muscle spindles. The spindles send sensorial signals to the spinal cord, informing the central nervous system (CNS) about the level of muscle contraction.

The CNS triggers nerve impulses that travel along the motor neuron toward the muscle fiber so that contraction can happen. They can excite the neuronal membrane to reach depolarization voltage levels above a triggering threshold that generates a particular wave known as action potential (AP). The AP consistently propagates along the axon toward the synaptic ending. At the synaptic cleft, vesicles deliver the neurotransmitter acetylcholine that connects to cholinergic receptors and depolarizes the myoneural junction. Eventually, the depolarization can generate a new AP that propagates along the sarcolemma leading to muscle contraction. In this process, fibers can stretch, shorten, or remain isometric although producing force. This force, in turn, is transmitted to the tendinous and bony structures [1]. Movement occurs that way. All these forms of motricity work well for a healthy subject. However, everything changes when spinal cord injury (SCI) occurs. **Figure 1** illustrates the central nervous system and its afferent and efferent pathways.

People with SCI have ruptured or impaired communication between CNS and organs that control motor and/or sensory functions. Nerve impulses are electrochemical processes and their transmissions occur in two directions. From CNS to PNS, they trigger muscle contraction processes. From PNS to CNS, they send sensorial processes that capture the stimuli from the surrounding environment as shown in **Figure 1** [1].

SCI harms the neurological responses according to the compromised site, that is, the level of the affected pathways. Thus, a complete SCI, which interrupts all nerve pathways, comprises in the acute-phase (also known as a medullary shock) flaccid paralysis with deep areflexia and muscle hypotonia to, consequently, give rise to spastic paralysis with hypertonia, deep hyperreflexia, and a sign of pyramidal release. Sensitive changes (hypoesthesia or anesthesia) occur for all forms of sensitivity below the level of injury. Partial or incomplete lesions are a consequence of the affected pathways. For instance, if there is a spinal hemisection, then there will be homolateral and contralateral signs and symptoms. On the same side of the injury, paresis or paralysis of the first neuron, abolition of deep sensations and alteration of gait occur. On the contralateral side, thermal and painful anesthesia is observed with no change in strength.

In the last decades, neuroscientists and rehabilitation engineers have been seeking alternatives to recover the mobility of people with SCI. The goal was to provide them with a better quality of life and functional independence. In 2012, the World Health Organization (WHO) asserted that about 0.5% of the population in developing countries needs prosthetic and orthotic devices and that 1.0% of that population needs wheelchairs [3]. Between 250,000 and 500,000 people suffer from SCI in the world, of which the majority are men and women between the ages of 15 and 25 and the elderly over 60 [4]. For the elderly, according to the United Nations Population Report [5], there will be an abrupt increase of people over 60 in 2050, reaching around 1 billion people among healthy individuals, people with SCI, heart

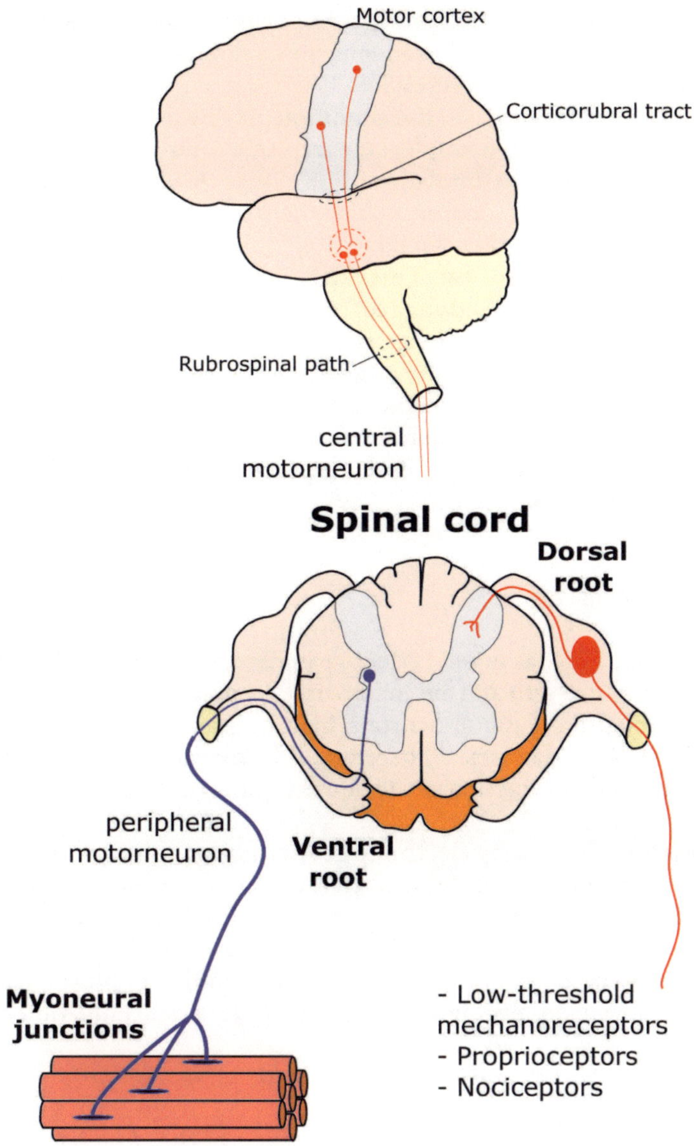

Figure 1.
Central nervous system and its afferent and efferent pathways [2].

disease, and other factors that may compromise locomotion. More than 1.2 million people in the United States have SCI that disables mobility, generating an estimated annual cost of $ 40.5 billion [6]. A Canadian study with 1716 individuals with SCI indicated a median lifetime expenditure of $ 336,000 per person, up to $ 479,000 if bedsores occur early in the hospital [7]. As costs are high, new techniques and devices are researched and evaluated to reduce these costs and/or minimize the impacts caused by immobility.

Devices such as wheelchairs, crutches, and walkers have been in use to aid the locomotion and rehabilitation of the elderly or people with SCI. However, these solutions are not fully effective and users expend great energy. It also requires the assistance of physiotherapists, caregivers, or family members [8, 9]. Therefore, alternatives that reduce the physical demands of users, therapists, and caregivers have been sought. Orthoses, neuroprostheses, and exoskeletons emerged as technologies that assist the individual's general health and therapeutic rehabilitation. These devices are capable of producing more intense training, quantitative feedback, and better functional results [9, 10].

In the case of people with SCI, the condition may be irreversible, resulting in some type of paresis: partial hemiplegia, paraplegia, or quadriplegia. Orthoses and/or functional electrical stimulation (FES) allow those people to perform ambulation (active orthoses) and/or provide them trunk stability (passive orthoses). Such technologies facilitate their social reintegration, increase self-esteem, and improve the general quality of life. This can be achieved since these solutions induce a decrease in other affections caused by limb paralysis, such as muscular atrophy, which reduces muscle strength and can prevent functional movements from happening [11–13]. Among the other sequelae that may arise as a consequence of SCI, one can mention: respiratory difficulties, intestinal and/or urinary incontinence, loss of sexual functions, deficiency of lymphatic and vascular system, muscle atrophy (which can result in spasticity), pressure ulcers, thrombosis, and bone demineralization [14].

2. Neuroprosthesis

Since the 1970s, FES has proved effective in restoring functional movements for both increasing strength and aid in impaired locomotion. It is being applied as a means of excitation of motor neurons. In SCI subjects, it bypasses the injury and bridges the CNS and muscles. Therefore, FES can cause real movement with an artificially evoked contraction as the injured spinal cord has this compromised communication [1, 15].

The bypass is performed by electronic devices known as functional electrical stimulators. The stimulators apply an electric current to the neuromuscular tissue through either implanted or non-implanted electrodes. In general, they consist of a pulse generator circuit or modulator (low voltage—up to 12 V), an amplifier (which increases voltage—up to 250 V) that provides the stimulatory pulses to be applied, and an isolated power supply. **Figure 2** illustrates a generic stimulation system.

2.1 Modulation (pulse generation)

Pulse generators determine the essential features of the stimulatory pulse, such as frequency, duration, and waveform. Many technologies have been used over time as innovations emerged in electronic devices. The pulse generator of a

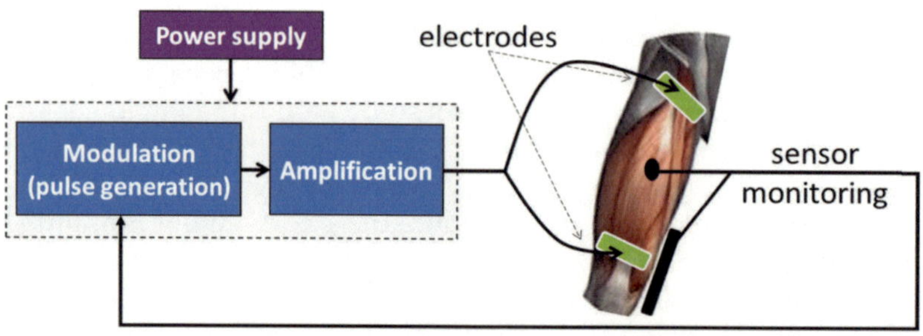

Figure 2.
Block diagram of a single-channel functional electrical stimulator. The essential steps for FES-elicited contraction involve the generation, amplification, and application of these pulses to the neuromuscular tissue. Sensors can help to correct pulse parameters as well as to determine the triggering time. All modules require power supply, whereas sensors may be active or passive.

functional electrical stimulator used two multivibrators, one configured as monostable and the other as astable, based on the LM555 integrated circuit (IC) [16]. Subsequent attempts, in turn, used development boards and more advanced digital components. One equipment used a Texas Instruments TMS320C32 digital signal processor (DSP) to control and generate arbitrary waveforms and to manage the stimulator [17]. The Arduino platform was employed and the ATMEL® microcontroller adjusted the stimulatory pulse frequency by means of a digital potentiometer [18]. Alternatively, others implemented a pulse generation module in a Motorola 68HC11F1™ microcontroller [19]. Generally, the stimulation parameters of a neuroprosthesis are generated and adapted by control algorithms that receive data from walking sensors and allow adaptation to a user's walking speed.

Use of ICs specifically designed for functional rehabilitation with the very large scale of integration (VLSI) has been growing rapidly. A common approach for pulse generation is to use a simple and inexpensive microcontroller for each stimulus output channel. A PIC16F84 microcontroller was used exclusively as a pulse generator [20]. The pulse formatting was performed via a virtual graphical interface. More recently, a solution used a virtual module for pulse generation. It was implemented in a virtual control instrument connected to a data acquisition and control board [21].

In order to achieve the most efficient biomechanical task and meet the appropriate physiological conditions, stimulatory pulses are modulated. This process changes the original waveform depending on the shape or value of a second signal. The resulting signal is indeed the mathematical composition of the previous ones. Pulse amplitude, duration, and frequency modulation facilitate access to more or less deep neuromotor units. Pulse amplitude modulation (PAM) and pulse width modulation (PWM) are the most frequent techniques [22]. PWM allows the energy delivered to the biological load to be controlled.

Stimulatory waveforms can be rectangular or exponential in shape, have a pulse width ranging from 0.01 to 1 ms, and burst frequency from 20 up to 100 Hz. Possible pain sensation is related to the transfer of electric charge from the stimulator to the user. Pulse durations between 100 and 300 μs cause little heat dissipation in the application area, leading to lower levels of pain [23]. Values shorter than 10 μs reduce the risk of intramuscular damage and those between 64 and 1230 μs can cause small skin irritation. The minimum burst contraction frequency is 10 Hz; however, apparent muscle tremor can be observed. Tremor is imperceptible with 30-Hz burst frequency. Muscle relaxation occurs from 300 to 700 Hz. There is less skin irritation with 2-kHz pulse frequency modulated at 50 Hz and lasting 10 ms [23].

For a muscle contraction to occur, a single pulse frequency can be selected between 20 and 400 Hz. However, the frequency considered optimal for force production ranges from 2.5 to 5 kHz, with burst frequency from 150 to 500 Hz, and pulse width from 10 to 30% of the duty cycle. Despite this, studies indicate that pain levels can get considerably high. To minimize the painful perception, frequencies between 9 and 10 kHz are more adequate, although they do not provide the same muscle strength [23, 24].

One of the widely used wave patterns is the so-called Russian current. Pulse frequency is 2.5 kHz, with 50-Hz bursts, 10-ms per train duration, and 10-ms intervals [24].

2.2 Amplification stage

The second most important stage when building an electrical stimulation device is amplification. This module consists of an arrangement of electronic components for commuting voltage or current signals. These circuit components shape signals accordingly to stimulate the neuromuscular tissue. A matter of the highest concern is

Type of motor unit	Contraction velocity	Fatigue resistance	Force
Slow	Slow	High	Low
Fatigue resistant	Fast	Intermediary	Intermediary
Fast fatigable	Fast	Low	High

Table 1.
Motor units and their features.

user safety. Amplification usually involves safety precautions since it is the last stage in the signal chain to be in contact with the user's skin and tissues through leads and electrodes. There are two modes to apply current to neuromuscular tissue: constant voltage or constant current. The difference is that current intensity depends on biological and interface impedances in the former but not in the latter. Determining this feature implies choosing a particular topology for the output circuit [25].

Current can flow in and out of the tissue depending on the signal reference. The allowed reference signals demand appropriate output stages. Depending on the reference, the current waveform can be monophasic or biphasic. Monophasic outputs allow only unidirectional current flow. This current waveform creates charge imbalances in the tissue. Conversely, biphasic outputs allow applying to and taking electrical charges out of the tissue. This bidirectional current flow prevents charge accumulation. This phenomenon is harmful to the subject for it can cause chemical burns mainly around the application site [26].

FES equipment can have one or more stimulatory output stages, usually called channels, each one responsible for the stimulation of a different muscle. For gait applications, usually, multichannel FES equipment is necessary to evoke more natural movements.

The motor neuron must be intact for FES application, otherwise there will be no muscle contraction. Thus, SCI type and level determine the use or avoidance of this technology.

Another issue to consider is the muscle to be stimulated. Each muscle is formed by a specific fiber type. When excited, the motor units contract at distinct speeds and resistance to muscle fatigue, delimiting the generation of force [1]. These features can be observed in **Table 1**.

3. Hybrid neuroprosthesis

Focus on technologies that bring users functional independence is increasing and, therefore, FES devices and active orthoses are thriving. In the previous session, the neuroprostheses were described in terms of their basic principle of operation and main characteristics. Like conventional prostheses and orthoses, neuroprostheses have advantages and disadvantages compared to other techniques when it comes to generating movement. Choosing a particular neuroprosthesis may depend on the severity of the user's condition, the type of task and the performance to be obtained, the cost of acquisition and maintenance as well as durability and energy efficiency.

Employed individually, a conventional orthosis has a large physical demand on the upper limbs and its energy cost is quite high [27]. As the upper limbs have a limited range for ambulation, gait patterns obtained with this technique are inappropriate. Over time, users stop using such orthoses to perform functional tasks and end up using them only for therapeutic purposes [28].

Initially, neuromuscular electrical stimulation served to compensate for muscle atrophy or counterbalance the effects of spasticity. The first efforts in the application of electrical stimulation with functional purposes began with the attempt to maintain a person with SCI in the orthostatic position, through the production of isometric tetanic muscle contractions, as originally proposed by Bajd et al. [29]. The attempt to ambulate using neuroprostheses followed and now it is possible to find many applications using FES to perform joint movements [30]. The main advantage of FES over conventional orthoses is that the muscle itself works as the supporting structure and the motor that propels the intended movements. The disadvantage, however, is that during FES sessions, rapid installation of muscle fatigue occurs. The depletion of metabolic resources becomes an obstacle to ambulation for long distances and it hampers the fine control of joint angle trajectories [31]. The control strategies of electrical stimulation combined with invasive electrodes have been proposed to minimize the well-known disadvantages of using FES.

Robotic systems have been receiving increasing attention from both health science and engineering researchers. This is due to the various possibilities of use and locomotor training. Some examples are the LOKOMAT® system that assists people with SCI to perform walking, through mimicking human gait on a treadmill, and the active orthoses that not only mimic gait but also give such people the freedom to move around the environment and sit/stand, walk, and climb/descend stairs [32]. These orthoses are wearable devices. They have (motor, hydraulic, or pneumatic) actuators parallel to the hip, knee, and ankle joints. They can only mimic the gait with the aid of mechanical devices that limit or expand the joint degrees of freedom. This makes the gait robotic in appearance and the actuators consume a lot of power, thus considerably reducing the system's autonomy, limiting the user's independence and its application for the recovery of compromised movements [33, 34].

Although a technological solution that demanded a high degree of creativity in its development, the active orthosis produces a gait process in which the patient is only a passive element. There are no important direct physiological benefits to the paralyzed muscles during their use, but passive mobility. In contrast, FES has many physiological benefits such as the improvement of muscle tone and blood circulation in paralyzed limbs, the prevention of pressure ulcers, respiratory and/or urinary problems, and the reduction of spasticity among others [9, 12, 14]. However, the intense, long, and non-selective contraction causes the muscles to be unable to maintain the force for long periods. That is because muscle fatigue is installing and hampering the maintenance of the movement stability, denoting, therefore, limitation in the control over the movement as well as the time of use [12].

In this context, hybrid neuroprostheses (HNPs) are interesting because they combine FES with other techniques to perform functional movements. Particularly, systems that combine FES and orthoses have been introduced in the literature. This hybrid approach opens the way for the elaboration of strategies that focus on the advantages of each individual technique. Quite often in this combination set, the power applied for the occurrence of movement is provided by the electrical stimulator and the structure of the orthosis serves to stabilize the movement.

4. Hybridization of neuroprosthesis for the lower limbs

This session presents some hybrid applications of neuroprosthesis. It indicates joint control technologies, main control elements, and control strategy.

The first studies identified consisted of simulations of hybrid control systems. The device involved an active orthosis containing actuators in the hip, knee and ankle joints, angle and angular velocity sensors, and a conventional FES system. The whole system was controlled in a closed loop, using both biomechanical and dynamic equations to perform gait movements [35]. According to the results, simulations allow the reproduction of gait although studies with volunteers with real system and setting would still be required.

Researchers developed and evaluated an HNP based on a variable-impedance knee mechanism [36]. It regulates knee flexion to overcome the challenges of controlling eccentric contractions. This mechanism consists of a four-bar linkage with a magnetorheological damper, hip and knee hydraulic actuators. The solution reduced the amount of stimulation required for walking and could restore biologically correct knee motion. It locks the knee joint motion and, during the stance phase of gait, it supports the body against collapse. The association with an FES unit by means of a finite state machine (FSM) controller allowed the body forward. Heel contact detectors and joint angle sensors controlled the knee motion during stance and swing phases. Tests compared the HNP and only FES application. HNP decreased the load response by up to 40% in knee extensors.

Pressurized hydraulic fluid from an accumulator was also tried to supply energy to an HNP instead of electric motors [37]. The hydraulic drive provided adjustable assistive torque to an exoskeletal hip joint beyond the possibilities of FES systems. The volume of valves was controlled in both directions, which allowed the estimation of hip flexion angle. Springs and a clutch system provided the knee-locking capability.

The same research group built a muscle-driven controllable exoskeleton to restore walking, sitting, and standing to people with SCI [38]. They combined the mechanics used in [36] and adaptations to the hip control described in [37]. An external controller that reads embedded sensor signals and determines the appropriate adjustments to a finite state machine drives an implanted FES unit. The state machine commands and synchronizes both the exoskeleton and the stimulator. Users choose the desired functions by a wireless switch controller. Although implanted devices demand surgical intervention, they were able to restore the stepping function to three subjects. This HNP supports stair descent patterns, overcoming a task that is hardly achieved with only FES.

An active orthosis had knee and ankle joint actuators and an FES system [9]. A central controller adjusted FES parameters using two closed loops and six stimulation channels. Gait consists of two phases: balance and support. It uses FES during the balance phase and the orthosis is active during the support phase, which is the moment of gait that demands more energy expenditure from the patient. The solution presents the clear strategy of shortening the time interval between FES activations. This way, there will be more time for muscle recovery and, consequently, fewer episodes of fatigue over time. With the activation of the active orthosis, the system does not stay connected all the time and, thus, the energy demand of the system decreases.

Figure 3 shows a diagram that represents a hybrid neuroprosthesis. It consists of an electric stimulator and an active orthosis with actuators in its joints, feedback sensors for gait, and a real-time control system. This control system identifies the gait phases, evaluates the current position of the lower limbs, makes decisions to activate the actuators, or triggers the FES unit.

The controller is the main component. Gait takes place safely and naturally depending on how robust the interaction with mechanical parts is and how fast it reacts after receiving feedback information. Thus, increasing the feedback information volume may be an impacting differential between existing orthoses. More degrees of freedom per joint allow a more natural gait and this is an important factor. However, in the case of people with SCI, using only one degree of freedom per joint brings greater stability and safety during movement, thus avoiding joint injuries [33, 34].

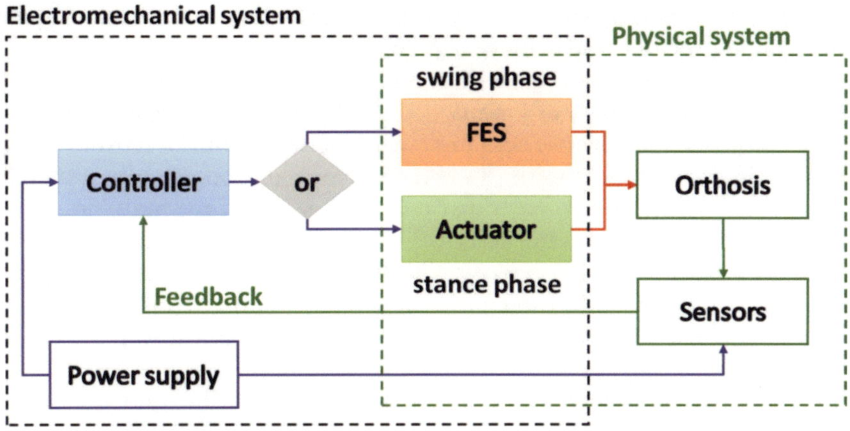

Figure 3.
Basic diagram of a hybrid neuroprosthesis system. It demonstrates the integration of the control system with the FES unit, actuators, and feedback sensors.

A semi-active hybrid orthosis [39] employed electric motors to actuate on hip movement whereas FES actuated on knee and ankle movements. Wrap spring clutches combine high torque capacity and millisecond response time. Their use prevented the knee flexion when they were locked while still holding the torque in one direction (knee extension). This approach eliminated the need for FES application during standing and to the stance leg during a step, saving muscle metabolic energy. Researchers intend to incorporate an FES channel in future HNP versions to stimulate the peroneal nerve and provide redundant actuation at the hip joint.

Another approach combined a commercial FES unit (RehaStim 2, Hasomed, Germany) and a knee exoskeleton for controlling knee joint swinging movements [40]. The main contribution is that the interactive forces of this solution are measurable and it helps in better cooperative control. The continuous decrease in muscle force performance is an indication of muscle fatigue installation. Therefore, the torque required to perform a task is distributed between both actuators (muscles under FES and electrical motor). Two interactive force sensors that measure the mutual force between exoskeleton and shank accomplish force readings. Each interactive force sensor provides equivalent summed value from six previously calibrated force-sensing resistors.

A cycling-induced HNP implemented a repetitive learning controller that allows uncertain, non-linear cycle-rider systems to track the desired cadence [41]. The controller feedback depended on the crank angle. FES applied to lower limb muscle groups drives the movements, whereas the electric motors come into play when stimulated muscles yield low torque values. The system tried to track the cadence of five able-bodied subjects and three subjects with neurological conditions. The results presented low root mean square errors.

Some devices are still in enhancement. An HNP consisted of orthotic components (reciprocating gait orthosis and rigid ankle-foot orthosis), powered backdrivable knee joints (obtained with custom harmonic drive transmissions and brushless DC motors), and was intended for use with FES [42]. One of the main contributions of this work was to be able to execute movements with a lightweight device, up to 10 kg.

Another attempt was the development of a 17.05-kg HNP prototype for short-range walking [43]. This device consists of a quadriceps single-channel FES unit and a passive energy-storing exoskeleton. Gas spring stores energy during knee extension and it delivers to knee and hip joint control when completing the gait cycle. Its walking speed could achieve 0.27 m/s.

The Research Group of the Rehabilitation Engineering Laboratory of the Pontifical Catholic University of Paraná (PUCPR) has also developed an active lower limb orthosis with electric actuators with angular feedback sensors in the hip and knee joints to perform gait [34, 44, 45]. Normally, an orthotic system has actuators in their joints, which are transverse to the joints of the individual who is "wearing" it, which facilitates the design of the system. Thus, the mechanical hip joint has a 26° flexion and a 13° extension limited by mechanical stops, as shown in **Figure 4** (1) [34]. Knee flexion and extension are in the range from 0° to 90°. The controller output will obey these limits as well as the mechanical stops, as shown in **Figure 4** (2).

Engines and transmissions will be coupled directly to the hip and knee joints, as shown in **Figure 4** (3 and 4). The gear ratio in the planetary-type transmission system is 4.75:1; so, the torque at the joint output will be 4.7 times larger than the engine torque [34].

For the control, it is necessary that there is an angular sensor in each joint, each one coupled to the axis of the motor by means of pulleys and synchronizing belt. In this way, it is possible to make the angle reading directly and in real time. Its structure with a partial weight support system can be seen in **Figure 5** [34].

The controller of the active orthosis synchronizes both knee and hip joints. A state machine simulates the gait phases and determines when each joint will engage, as shown in the diagram of **Figure 6**.

The control of each joint has predefined set points that correspond to the maximum and minimum angles of a healthy gait. It receives voltage readings of the angle sensor, calculates the actuating error, adjusts the PWM mathematically, and sends it to the motor drive. The error is determined as the difference between input angular value and angle sensor reading on the motor axis. The readings of angular sensors vary according to motor rotation. This may increase or decrease the error.

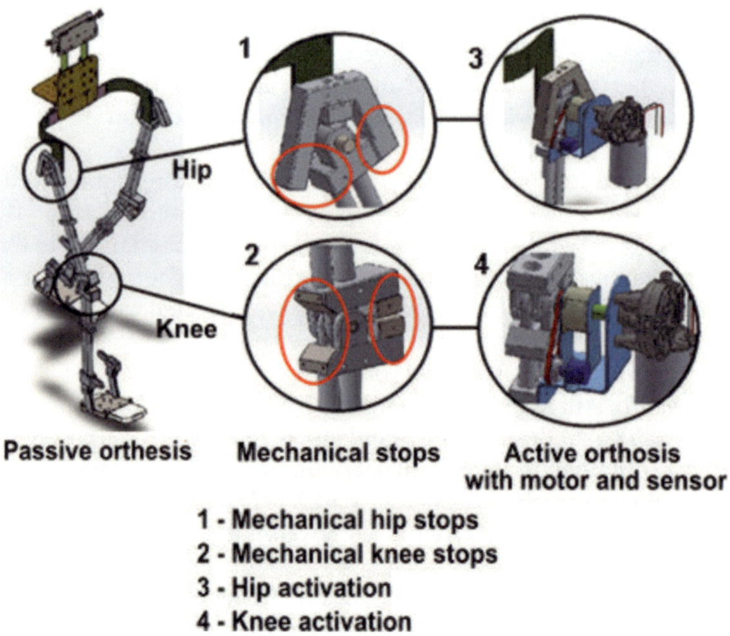

Figure 4.
Mechanical structure of the passive orthosis and activation sequence of actuators in the hip and knee joints.

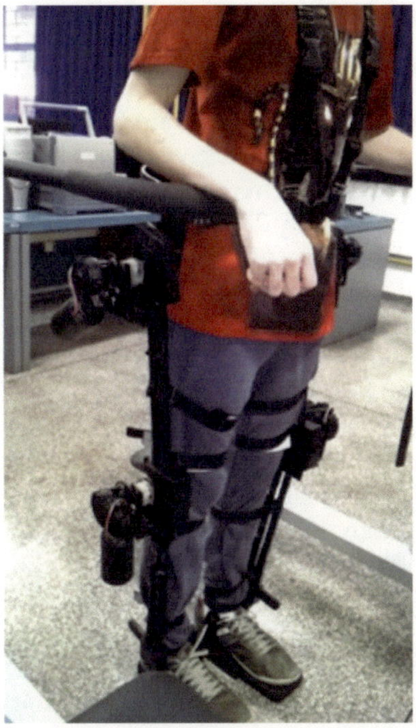

Figure 5.
Mechanical structure of the active orthosis with a volunteer on the partial weight support system.

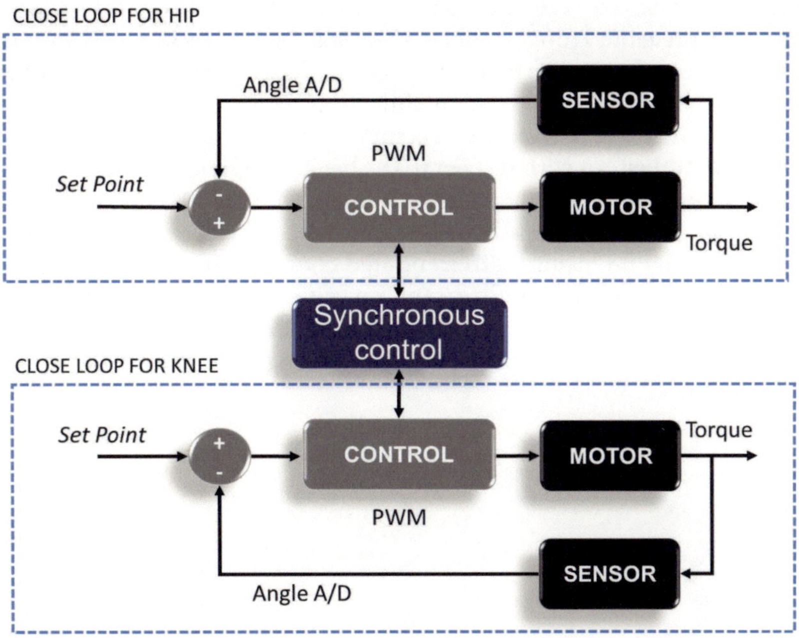

Figure 6.
Control block diagram of the active orthosis. Two loops operate synchronously to generate appropriate torque to hip and knee joints.

The closer the angle sensor reading is to the determined set point, the smaller the error. Consequently, because the motor is proportional to the driving error, the lower is the motor speed [34].

The results of active orthosis control tests, without volunteers, were normalized using MATLAB™ software (**Figure 7**) in comparison to the gait of a healthy individual (**Figures 8** and **9**) [34].

Figure 8 allows the observation of important factors. The maximum knee flexion angle achieves 50°. There is a difference presented as an initial flexion between 0 and 40% of the gait cycle, which appears in the dashed graph of the healthy individual with the amplitude of approximately 20°. The divergence is due to the reference point difference at which the angle was obtained, a bending that occurs in relation to the global system. Such lag exists because of the empirical way in which the control data are normalized. It is also because the hip could only flex and is limited to 26°, whereas knees could flex and extend. Therefore, there is a difference between the gait cadence of the developed system and the healthy gait. The former is faster than the latter. Nevertheless, the control will apply a 4.7:1 reduction in this speed, slowing down 4 times, making the orthosis cadence slower than a healthy one.

Another observation is that the healthy knee's initial angle is zero and this is due to the calibration of the system. If signals were stapled to have the same reference, the maximum bending angle would be less than 50°. This is because the control set points of the orthosis for people with SCI were adjusted to be lower than that of a healthy individual. Therefore, the control program should not allow angles to exceed the biomechanical limits equal to those of a healthy one.

Considering hip angle analysis, there were also angular differences due to the mechanical limits of the bracing. Hip flexion is limited to 26° and extension limited to 13°. In **Figure 9**, the negative half-cycle of the amplitude of the signal represents the hip extension.

Once again, the programmed angles were not limited to the maximum normal hip values, which worked as activation thresholds to the electronic safety circuit. This alternative prevented movements that exceed the biomechanical limits of the user using the orthosis. The control operation depends on the percent of gait. Consequently, the controlled movement duration is shorter than the gait of a healthy individual since the angle of movement is smaller. The solid line also denotes higher speed and sharp transition with respect to the healthy individual. However, once again, there is a 4.7:1 reduction in the speed, smoothing the gait cadence.

Studies with this system are still ongoing. One of the efforts is the hybridization of the orthosis with FES, using a differentiated control, so that there is a possible reduction in the energetic expenditure and muscular fatigue. The embedded strategy difference is to keep the hip joint under control throughout the gait and apply FES to knee extensor muscles only during gait swing phase. **Figure 10** presents the proposed system.

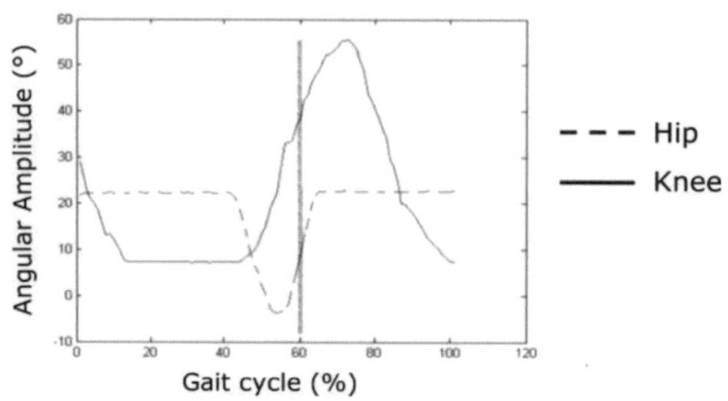

Figure 7.
Angular variation of both hip and knee joints (interval of one gait cycle).

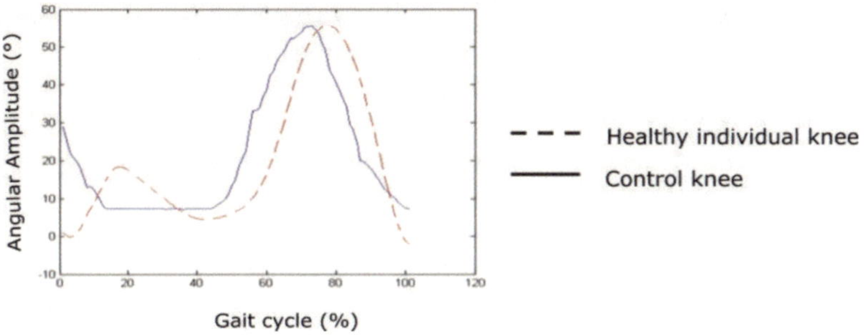

Figure 8.
Comparison of knee angular variation between orthosis control and healthy individual (interval of one gait cycle).

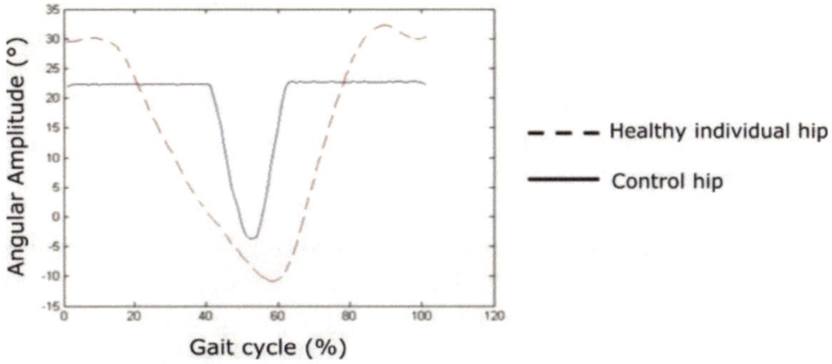

Figure 9.
Comparison of knee angular variation between orthosis control and healthy individual (interval of one gait cycle).

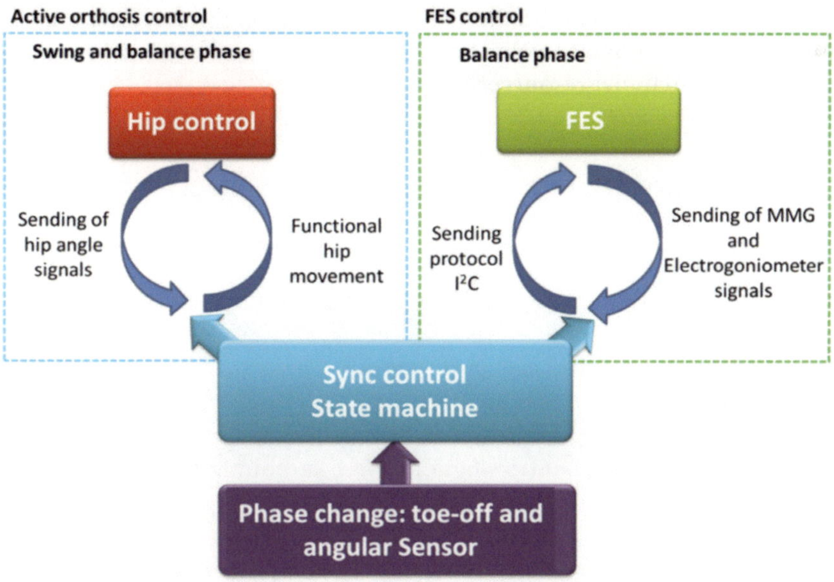

Figure 10.
Controller scheme with mechanomyography (MMG) and joint angle feedback at each stage of the gait.

Using the orthosis during both gait phases lessens the weight of the whole system on the user. In existing systems, when FES activates the muscles, the user has to raise both the mechanical apparatus and the limb. This weight-bearing requirement hastens the installation of muscle fatigue [9, 14] although it is smaller in relation to other systems that use only FES, or FES with passive orthosis [33].

This HNP has a fatigue detection system that processes mechanomyography signals [15]. The goal is to identify signal pattern changes and, in case of fatigue installation conditions, the HNP will activate the joint motors, guaranteeing user's safety.

Hybrid systems for locomotion using FES and active orthoses are relatively new devices. Despise this, there are a few projects addressing this aspect, which are enough to visualize and glimpse the benefits and perspectives of these technologies.

5. Conclusions

This chapter presented the principles of the neural prosthesis and discussed the reasons for the hybridization of these systems. The methods used to stimulate the muscles and develop a neuroprosthesis remain valid and the stimulatory parameters are the same. Researchers, however, use new embedded systems technologies and graphical interfaces to program and configure the internal parameters of FES equipment, also using hybridization of orthosis and neuroprosthesis to combine the advantages of individual techniques to counterbalance their individual disadvantages. The joint use of FES and orthosis attempts to reduce user's energy expenditure, postpone muscle fatigue installation, increase posture and movement stability, and reduce the system energy costs. Thus, hybrid neural prostheses increase system efficiency and prolong the time of use, consequently, achieving health benefits.

Acknowledgements

The authors would like to thank the National Council for Scientific and Technological Development (CNPq) and Araucária Foundation (FA) for the scholarships and financial resources.

Author details

Percy Nohama*, Guilherme Nunes Nogueira Neto and Maira Ranciaro
Pontifícia Universidade Católica do Paraná, Curitiba, Brazil

*Address all correspondence to: percy.nohama@pucpr.br

References

[1] Sweeney JD. In: Reilly JP, Hermann A, editors. Skeletal muscle response to electrical stimulation, Applied Bioelectricity. 1st ed. New York: Springer-Verlag; 1998. pp. 299-340

[2] Ordovas-Montanes J, Rakoff-Nahoum S, Huang S, Riol-Blanco L, Barreiro O, von Andrian UH. The regulation of immunological processes by peripheral neurons in homeostasis and disease. Trends in Immunology. 2015;**36**:578-604. DOI: 10.1016/j.it.2015.08.007

[3] WHO. Concept paper: WHO guidelines on health-related rehabilitation [Internet]. 2015. Available from: http://who.int/disabilities/care/rehabilitation_guidelines_concept.pdf [Accessed: 2018-09-10]

[4] WHO. Spinal cord injury [Internet]. 2013. Available from: http://www.who.int/mediacentre/factsheets/fs384/en/ [Accessed: 2018-09-10]

[5] UN. Population fact sheets: Population ageing and sustainable development [Internet]. 2014. Available from: http://www.un.org/en/development/desa/population/publications/pdf/popfacts/PopFacts_2014-4.pdf [Accessed: 2018-09-10]

[6] CDRF. Spinal cord injury [Internet]. 2016. [Accessed: 2018-09-10]

[7] Chan BC-F, Cadarette SM, Wodchis WP, Krahn MD, Mittmann N. The lifetime cost of spinal cord injury in Ontario, Canada: A population-based study from the perspective of the public health care payer. The Journal of Spinal Cord Medicine. 2018:1-10. DOI: 10.1080/10790268.2018.1486622

[8] Rupal B, Singla A, Virk G. Lower limb exoskeletons: A brief review. In: Conference on Mechanical Engineering and Technology (COMET-2016); Varanasi, India. IIT (BHU). 2016. pp. 130-140

[9] del-Ama AJ, Gil-Agudo Á, Pons JL, Moreno JC. Hybrid FES-robot cooperative control of ambulatory gait rehabilitation exoskeleton. Journal of Neuroengineering and Rehabilitation. 2014;**11**:27. DOI: 10.1186/1743-0003-11-27

[10] Chen G, Chan CK, Guo Z, Yu H. A review of lower extremity assistive robotic exoskeletons in rehabilitation therapy. Critical Reviews in Biomedical Engineering. 2013;**41**:343-363. DOI: 10.1615/CritRevBiomedEng.2014010453

[11] Fougeyrollas P, Noreau L. Long-term consequences of spinal cord injury on social participation: The occurrence of handicap situations. Disability and Rehabilitation. 2000;**22**:170-180. DOI: 10.1080/096382800296863

[12] del-Ama AJ, Koutsou AD, Moreno JC, de-los-Reyes A, Gil-Agudo A, Pons JL. Review of hybrid exoskeletons to restore gait following spinal cord injury. Journal of Rehabilitation Research and Development. 2012;**49**:497

[13] Sabut SK, Lenka PK, Kumar R, Mahadevappa M. Effect of functional electrical stimulation on the effort and walking speed, surface electromyography activity, and metabolic responses in stroke subjects. Journal of Electromyography and Kinesiology. 2010;**20**:1170. DOI: 10.1016/j.jelekin.2010.07.003

[14] Ha KH, Murray SA, Goldfarb M. An approach for the cooperative control of FES with a powered exoskeleton during level walking for persons with paraplegia. IEEE Transactions on Neural Systems and Rehabilitation Engineering. 2016;**24**:455-466. DOI: 10.1109/TNSRE.2015.2421052

[15] Nohama P, Krueger E, Nogueira-Neto GN, Scheeren E. Novas tecnologias para a reabilitação após lesão medular. In: Vall J, editor. Lesão Medular: Reabilitação e Qualidade de Vida. 1st ed. Rio de Janeiro: Atheneu; 2014. pp. 235-273

[16] Cheng KE, Lu Y, Tong K-Y, Rad AB, Chow DH, Sutanto D. Development of a circuit for functional electrical stimulation. IEEE Transactions on Neural Systems and Rehabilitation Engineering. 2004;**12**:43-47. DOI: 10.1109/TNSRE.2003.819936

[17] Wu H-C, Young S-T, Kuo T-S. A versatile multichannel direct-synthesized electrical stimulator for FES applications. IEEE Transactions on Instrumentation and Measurement. 2002;**51**:2-9. DOI: 10.1109/19.989882

[18] Johnsen E, DiMeo G, Franco B, Wilson R. Design and construction of an electrical muscle stimulation system to decrease Forearm Muscle Atrophy post-fracture. In: 37th Annual Northeast Bioengineering Conference (NEBEC); Troy. IEEE. 2011. pp. 1-2. DOI: 10.1109/nebc.2011.5778539

[19] O'Keeffe DT, Lyons GM. A versatile drop foot stimulator for research applications. Medical Engineering & Physics. 2002;**24**:237-242. DOI: 10.1016/S1350-4533(02)00011-5

[20] Laguna ZV, Cardiel E, Garay LI, Hernández PR. Electrical stimulator for surface nerve stimulation by using modulated pulses. In: 2011 Pan American Health Care Exchanges; Rio de Janeiro. IEEE. 2011. pp. 77-82. DOI: 10.1109/pahce.2011.5871852

[21] Velloso JB, Souza MN. A programmable system of functional electrical stimulation (FES). In: 29th Annual International Conference of the IEEE Engineering in Medicine and Biology Society; Lyon. IEEE. 2007. pp. 2234-2237. DOI: 10.1109/IEMBS.2007.4352769

[22] Hart DW. Power Electronics. New York: McGraw-Hill; 2011

[23] Webster JG. Electronic Devices for Rehabilitation. Hoboken: John Wiley & Sons Incorporated; 1985

[24] Tribioli RA. Análise crítica atual sobre a TENS envolvendo parâmetros de estimulação para o controle da dor [master dissertação]. Interunidades em Bioengenharia, São Carlos: Universidade de São Paulo; 2003

[25] Mottaghi S, Hofmann UG. Dynamically adjusted, scalable electrical stimulator for exciteable tissue. In: 7th International IEEE/EMBS Conference on Neural Engineering (NER); Montpellier. IEEE. 2015. pp. 288-291. DOI: 10.1109/NER.2015.7146616

[26] Xu Q, Huang T, He J, Wang Y, Zhou H. A programmable multi-channel stimulator for array electrodes in transcutaneous electrical stimulation. In: IEEE/ICME International Conference on Complex Medical Engineering (CME); Harbin Heilongjiang. IEEE. 2011. pp. 652-656. DOI: 10.1109/ICCME.2011.5876821

[27] Fatone S. A review of the literature pertaining to KAFOs and HKAFOs for ambulation. Journal of Prosthetics and Orthotics. 2006;**18**:P137-P168. DOI: 10.1097/00008526-200606001-00003

[28] Waters RL, Mulroy S. The energy expenditure of normal and pathologic gait. Gait & Posture. 1999;**9**:207-231. DOI: 10.1016/S0966-6362(99)00009-0

[29] Bajd T, Kralj A, Šega J, Turk R, Benko H, Strojnik P. Use of a two-channel functional electrical stimulator to stand paraplegic patients. Physical Therapy. 1981;**61**:526-527

[30] Peckham PH, Knutson JS. Functional electrical stimulation for neuromuscular applications. Annual Review of Biomedical Engineering.

2005;**7**:327-360. DOI: 10.1146/annurev.bioeng.6.040803.140103

[31] Thrasher TA, Popovic MR. Functional electrical stimulation of walking: Function, exercise and rehabilitation. Annales de Réadaptation et de Médecine Physique. 2008;**51**:452-460. DOI: 10.1016/j.annrmp.2008.05.006

[32] van Kammen K, Boonstra AM, van der Woude LHV, Reinders-Messelink HA, den Otter R. The combined effects of guidance force, bodyweight support and gait speed on muscle activity during able-bodied walking in the Lokomat. Clinical biomechanics. 2016;**36**:65-73. DOI: 10.1016/j.clinbiomech.2016.04.013

[33] Yang L, Condie DN, Granat MH, Paul JP, Rowley DI. Effects of joint motion constraints on the gait of normal subjects and their implications on the further development of hybrid FES orthosis for paraplegic persons. Journal of Biomechanics. 1996;**29**:217-226. DOI: 10.1016/0021-9290(95)00018-6

[34] Ranciaro M, Neto GNN, Fernandes CR, da Cunha JC, Nohama P. Mimetic motion control for a lower-extremity active orthosis for hemiplegic people. IEEE Latin America Transactions. 2017;**15**:225-231. DOI: 10.1109/TLA.2017.7854616

[35] Ohashi T, Obinata G, Shimada Y, Ebata K. Control of hybrid FES system for restoration of paraplegic locomotion. In: 2nd IEEE International Workshop on Robot and Human Communication; Tokyo. IEEE. 1993. pp. 96-101. DOI: 10.1109/ROMAN.1993.367741

[36] Bulea TC, Kobetic R, Audu ML, Schnellenberger JR, Triolo RJ. Finite state control of a variable impedance hybrid neuroprosthesis for locomotion after paralysis. IEEE Transactions on Neural Systems and Rehabilitation Engineering. 2013;**21**:141-151. DOI: 10.1109/tnsre.2012.2227124

[37] Foglyano KM, Kobetic R, To CS, Bulea TC, Schnellenberger JR, Audu ML, et al. Feasibility of a hydraulic power assist system for use in hybrid neuroprostheses. Applied Bionics and Biomechanics. 2015;**2015**:205104. DOI: 10.1155/2015/205104

[38] Chang SR, Nandor MJ, Li L, Kobetic R, Foglyano KM, Schnellenberger JR, et al. A muscle-driven approach to restore stepping with an exoskeleton for individuals with paraplegia. Journal of Neuroengineering and Rehabilitation. 2017;**14**:48. DOI: 10.1186/s12984-017-0258-6

[39] Kirsch N, Alibeji N, Fisher L, Gregory C, Sharma N. A semi-active hybrid neuroprosthesis for restoring lower limb function in paraplegics. In: 36th Annual International Conference of the IEEE Engineering in Medicine and Biology Society; IEEE. 2014. pp. 2557-2560. DOI: 10.1109/EMBC.2014.6944144

[40] Zhang D, Ren Y, Gui K, Jia J, Xu W. Cooperative control for a hybrid rehabilitation system combining functional electrical stimulation and robotic exoskeleton. Frontiers in Neuroscience. 2017;**11**:725. DOI: 10.3389/fnins.2017.00725

[41] Duenas VH, Cousin CA, Parikh A, Freeborn P, Fox EJ, Dixon WE. Motorized and functional electrical stimulation induced cycling via switched repetitive learning control. IEEE Transactions on Control Systems Technology. 2018. DOI: 10.1109/TCST.2018.2827334

[42] Weaver VA. Design and fabrication of a hybrid neuroprosthetic exoskeleton for gait restoration [master]. Department of Mechanical and Aerospace Engineering, Cleveland: Case Western Reserve University; 2017

[43] Katti VV. Design of a muscle-powered walking exoskeleton for

people with spinal cord injury [master]. Minnesota: University of Minnesota; 2018

[44] Ranciaro M. Controle mimético de marcha de um membro inferior para órtese ativa [master]. Health Technology, Curitiba: Pontifical Catholic University of Parana; 2016

[45] Fernandes CR, Fernandes BL, Ranciaro M, Stefanello J, Nohama P. Model proposal for development of a passive exoeskeleton for lower limb. In: V Congresso Brasileiro de Eletromiografia e Cinesiologia (COBEC); Uberlandia. SBEB. 2017. pp. 664-666. DOI: 10.29327/cobecseb.78856

Chapter 4

Residual Limb Health and Prosthetics

Sashwati Roy, Shomita S. Mathew-Steiner and Chandan K. Sen

Abstract

The residual limb of individuals with lower limb loss is dynamic tissue that is susceptible to both acute and chronic changes to limb volume and health over time. Changes in residual limb volume that affect socket fit may contribute to maladaptive gait patterns and deleterious changes to the socket/limb interface that increase harmful shear stress and contributes to residual limb skin injury. Current socket systems are static and lack the ability to provide end-users and prosthetists with patient-centric data about changes in socket fit over time. There is a need for objective clinical decision-making that results in greater prosthesis usage, improved residual limb health, and better comfort ratings for end-users. Among the socket systems available in the market, the elevated vacuum suspension system improves residual limb skin oxygenation, attenuates socket-induced reactive hyperemia and preserves skin barrier function. This suggests that such a system is compatible with imparting physiological benefits to the residual limb in people with lower limb amputations.

Keywords: amputation, prosthesis, residual limb health, transepidermal water loss, surface electrical capacitance, skin barrier, perfusion

1. Introduction

Prosthetics are artificial substitutes for body parts lost through congenital defects, injury (accident or combat-related) or disease. These devices can be worn on the outside of the body or surgically implanted and are made of a variety of materials that may serve a cosmetic and/or functional purpose. They have evolved from simple fiber-based appendages (ancient Egypt) to the sophisticated lower limb "blades" and bionic arms that enable amputees to transcend barriers to their activities. Prosthetics today are strong and light, made of aluminum, plastic or composite materials that are better molded to the patient limb. Furthermore, the advent of microprocessors, computer chips and robotic technology provide a range of motion that fits the lifestyle choices of the amputee.

Achieving a comfortable and functional connection between an amputee and their prosthetic limb is critical to the success of the prosthesis. Therefore, the socket system is the most significant component for overall success of the prosthesis [1, 2]. Plaster wraps or computer aided designs are the primary means to custom fit sockets to maximize socket performance and comfort without adversely affecting residual limb health (**Figure 1**). Currently, the lack of quantitative feedback to determine appropriate socket fit is a major drawback in this process. Prosthetists use anecdotal visual cues combined with subjective verbal feedback from patients to minimize suspension-dependent movement between the socket and residual limb. This subjective information is used to revise socket parameters such as volume, geometry, and type of suspension to provide a "best" fit for the amputee. In day-to-day living, the volume of mature residual limb (>18 months postamputation [3]) are subject to short-term [4] and long-term [5, 6] changes in volume that compromise socket fit and performance.

More than 80% of amputations in the U.S. are the result of complications from vascular disease and diabetes [7, 8]. Less than 10% of lower-limb amputation results from trauma [9]. In the US, among those that live with a lower-limb amputation, a growing number of which are Service men and women [10–12], the limb volume changes adversely affect fit, performance, and residual limb health [6]—including skin breakdown and ulceration [13] (**Figure 1**) that can require surgical revision of the amputation. The requirement for surgical revision is known to be as high as 30% [14]. This review primarily focuses on skin health in the residual lower limb and the need for objective monitoring and evaluation of changes at the interface of the biological entity (limb skin) and the artificial entity (prosthetic limb) for sustained optimal limb health. Similar issues could apply to the residual upper limb.

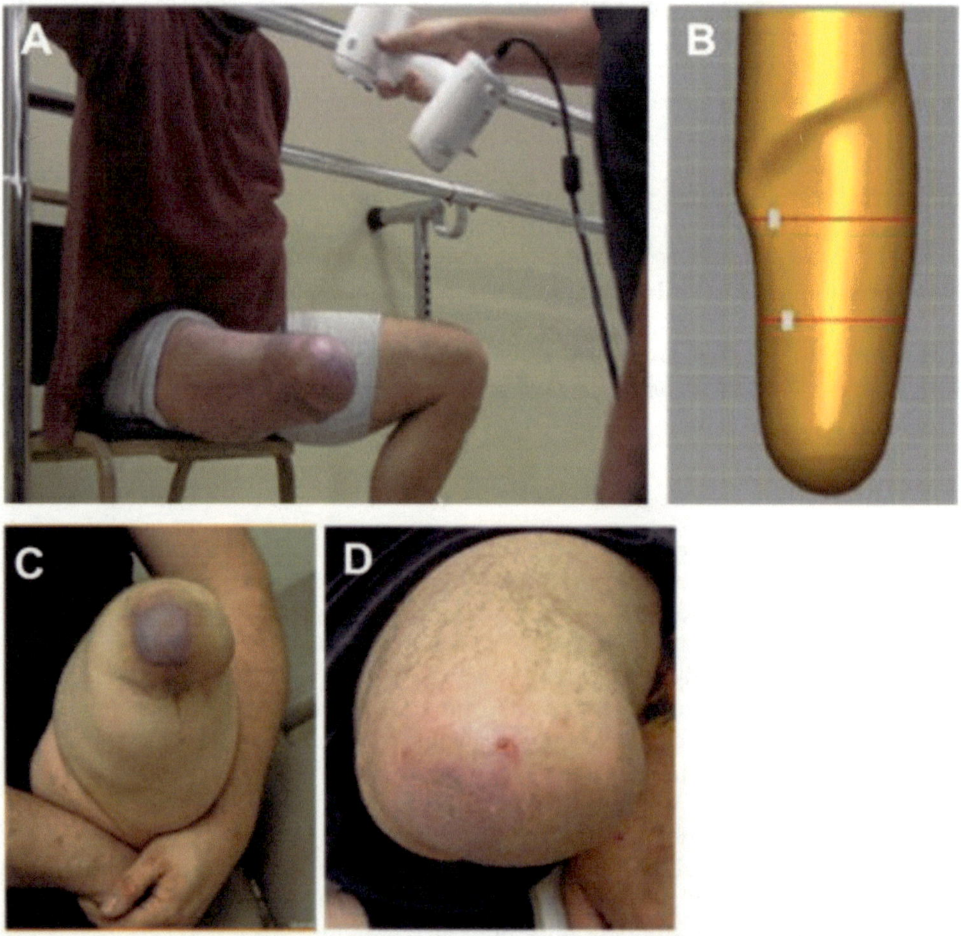

Figure 1.
(A) Prosthetists use a scanning device to digitize limb shape. (B) Digital model is modified to create a positive mold for socket fabrication tailored to the residual limb. (C) Tissue injury as a result of using a pin-locking suspension system. (D) Injury healed once the amputee was fit and began wearing an elevated vacuum suspension socket (EVS).

2. Overview of the prosthetic lower limb

2.1 Components

There are two main types of prosthetics that replace a partial or complete loss of the lower limb and these include: (a) below the knee or transtibial (TT), where a prosthetic lower leg is attached to an intact residual upper limb, (b) above the knee or transfemoral (TF), where a prosthesis replaces the upper and lower leg and knee. Each of these types of prostheses is composed of key parts: the prosthetic limb, a socket (interface between the biological component (e.g., patients' body) and the artificial limb), the attachments and the control system.

2.2 Socket systems

The piece that interfaces between the residual limb/body part and the artificial limb is called the socket and is typically molded around a plaster cast taken from the residual limb. A range of suspension systems are available for use on amputees and the choice of socket primarily depends on subjective information obtained by the prosthetist. The fit of a socket has to be precise or the artificial limb may cause discomfort or tissue damage resulting in the inability to wear the prosthesis for a time and leading to surgical interventions.

The most common systems in use are pin/shuttle lock, suction, and vacuum. The pin/lock system uses a padded liner with a pin on the end which is inserted into a shuttle lock built into the bottom of the connecting socket. A modification of this system is the lanyard, which connects the socket to the liner and limits shear and rotation. The suction system has a soft liner, a one-way valve and a sealing valve. Suction enables even adhesion to the interior surface of the socket and lowers the friction and shear. The vacuum system actively creates a seal around the socket and liner and enhances the adhesion of the limb to the socket, thereby regulating residual limb volume changes and promoting better circulation and reduced shear. The pin-lock is most popular but is associated with issues such as bell clapping (lateral displacement), pistoning (vertical displacement) (**Figure 2**) and distal tissue stretching (milking) which result in complications such as gait asymmetry, skin sores, and stump pain at the distal end. Suction and vacuum systems help minimize these complications and are currently popular (~95%) among Service Members and veterans with limb loss.

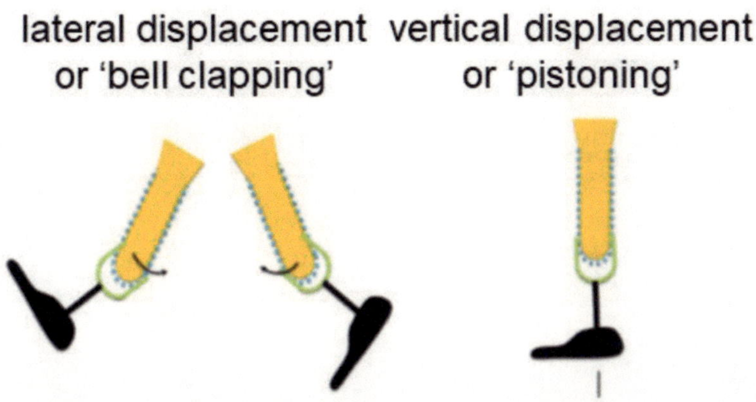

Figure 2.
Classification of residual limb movement within the socket. The timing and waveform profile are distinct in each of these types of movements.

2.3 The socket/limb interface

The importance of the socket/limb interface has been highlighted in several published reports. The primary concerns reported from prosthesis users include the fit of the artificial limb and comfort. A study by Klute et al., identified that the time-consuming prosthesis fitting process can contribute to excess pressure and friction on the residual limb, resulting in skin and deeper tissue damage and related pain and discomfort [15]. The outcome of this study emphasized the need for a fitting process that included objective measures to complement and improve user feedback.

Several studies employing radiological [15–17], acoustic [18], and optical [19] approaches have been used to analyze the movement of the residual limb within the socket of lower limb systems. These have numerous shortcomings primarily related to lack of clinical translatability and testing capability in a limited range of movements. The LimbLogic® vacuum system developed as a result of a Veterans Affairs (VA) grant funded collaborative work with Ohio Willow Wood was commercialized for clinically relevant quantification of prosthetic socket performance. Elevated vacuum suspension (EVS) [20, 21] (**Figure 3**) creates subatmospheric pressure between the prosthetic socket and liner worn over the residual limb. Studies performed with this system identified that variances among individuals may be a result of different gait styles, tissue types, residual limb geometries, prosthesis weight distribution, and socket fit. The results demonstrated that elevated vacuum pressure data provide information to quantify initial socket fit and monitor changes from an initial set point. The correlation between displacement and vacuum pressure fluctuation was dependent on socket fit. In general, higher vacuum pressure settings resulted in the lower amounts of displacement and vacuum pressure fluctuation within each socket fit condition. However, the rates of decreases created distinct trends in the data that correlated to particular fit conditions.

Therefore, the effectiveness of lower limb prosthesis is largely measured by its ability to minimize in-socket movement of the residual limb, conserving residuum health. Movement of the residual limb within the prosthetic socket contributes to increased risk of skin ulceration [22]. Technological advancements in residual limb scanning and socket manufacturing have empowered prosthetists to design and

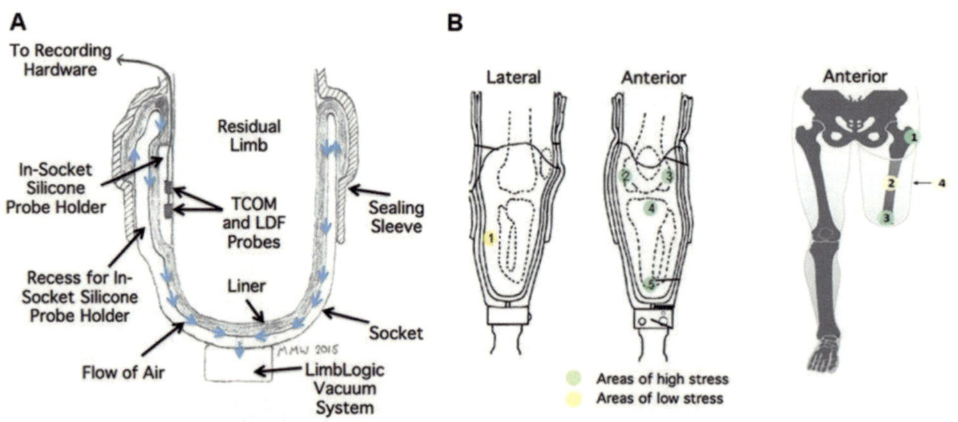

Figure 3.
Elevated vacuum suspension schematic and probe measurement points. (A) Illustration of test socket with recess for in-socket silicone probe holder. (B) Residual-limb measurement sites. Green and yellow indicate measurement sites of high and low stress, respectively. LDF = laser Doppler flowmetry, TCOM = transcutaneous oxygen measurement (reprinted with permission from Rink et al. [20]).

fit customized sockets that account for unique amputee residual limb shape and volume. However, unlike the rigid socket that is fixed in geometry and volume, the morphometry of the residual limb is dynamic. Mature residual limbs experience diurnal changes in volume of up to 2% [4] because of a number of factors including activity level, ambient environment, body composition, dietary habits, and hormones [6]. Furthermore, chronic remodeling of a mature residual limb can result in even greater (~10%) volume changes over the course of weeks [23] and months [5]. Thus, socket fit and residual limb movement in the socket are subject to time-dependent changes. Because socket movement increases risk of residuum dermal injury and ulceration [22], there is a clear need to evaluate the efficacy of using a socket monitoring system that can quantify residual limb movement inside the socket to aid in the socket fitting process. Such a system has the potential of minimizing risk to residual limb health [6] while maximizing functional performance.

3. Residual limb health

3.1 Issues with prosthesis fitting

Achieving a comfortable and functional connection between an amputee and their prosthetic limb is critical to the success of the prosthesis. Therefore, the socket system is the most significant component for the overall rehabilitative success of the prosthesis [24, 25]. Socket comfort is achieved by appropriately loading and off-loading the residual limb, where the optimal biomechanical performance of the prosthesis is achieved by transfer motions of the residual limb without loss or excess motion to the prosthesis. In an effort to maximize socket performance and comfort without adversely affecting residual limb health, a prosthetist custom fits a socket for every patient using plaster wraps or computer aided design. Currently, this process suffers from a lack of quantitative feedback to determine appropriate socket fit. Prosthetists aim to create a comfortable and intimate socket interface, but current approaches are limited as they rely on anecdotal visual cues along with subjective verbal feedback from the patient. Prosthetists then use this information to revise socket parameters such as volume, geometry, and type of suspension to provide a "best" fit for a patient.

In light of the subjective inputs that currently inform prosthesis form, fit, and therefore function, there is a clear need to provide objective measures to optimize prosthesis fitting and provide continual feedback to both end-user and prosthetist as the residual limb volume and shape are susceptible to change over time. Under the current paradigm of prosthetic socket fitting, inadequate and/or misinformation communicated to the prosthetist can lead to sub-optimal fit and comfort of the prosthetic system. This contributes to repeat clinical visits to rectify areas of discomfort, or in more extreme cases rejection of the prosthesis and preference toward other assistive devices such as wheelchairs. Two surveys administered to lower limb prosthesis users indicated a high prevalence of skin sores or irritation occurring within the socket, with fit likely being a contributing factor [24, 25]. If left unresolved, such limb health issues may necessitate disuse of the prosthesis.

3.2 Injuries of the residual limb

Most amputees have an active and satisfying quality of life with a majority that wear a prosthesis at least 7 h a day to aid in mobility and everyday living. An improper fit or alignment, lack of adequate gait training and development of poor habits are common features of a vast majority of amputees who use a prosthesis resulting in at least one deviation or problem. The increased load or weight is often placed on the intact limb as a result of these deviations can cause discomfort or pain in the joints and lead to some form of degenerative joint disease or disability in extreme cases. Three of the most common secondary complications in lower-limb amputees due to compensatory and/or altered stresses are osteoarthritis, osteoporosis and back pain.

About 75% of patients with lower-limb prosthetics have skin problems [26, 27]. The lack of a normal pressure-distributing anatomy the residual limb is prone to issues such as elevated shear forces, stress risers, increased humidity, and prolonged moist contact within the prosthesis, which can contribute to ulceration. Ulcers or pressure sores, are the most common skin conditions in prosthetic users [24]

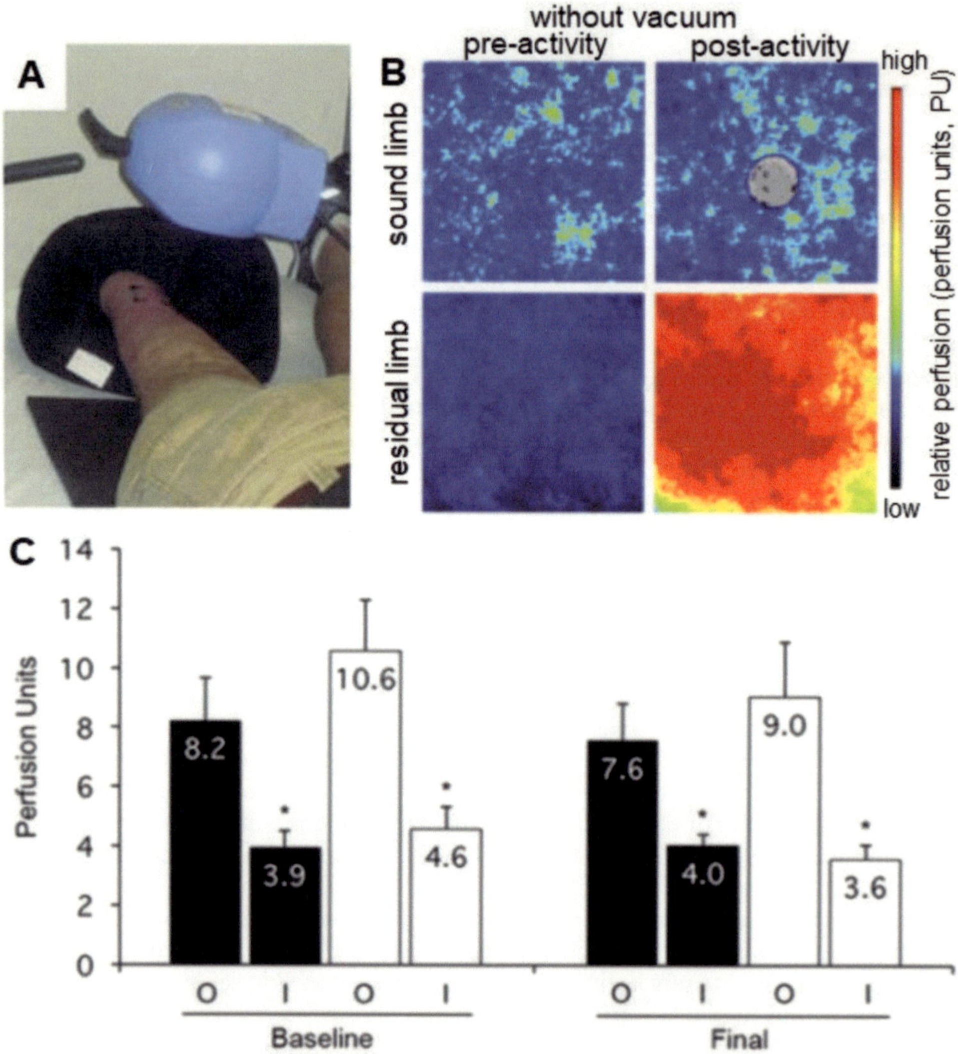

Figure 4.
*Laser speckle imaging (LSI) for skin perfusion. (A) Black box over transtibial amputee represents field of view (FOV) for perfusion mapping and quantification. (B) Representative perfusion maps acquired pre- and post-activity (over-ground walking) in sound and residual limb. (C) Perfusion was measured by laser Doppler flowmetry out-of-socket with liner on (O) and in-socket while resting with weight bearing on the residual limb (I) under SoC (black bar) and EVS (white bar) conditions. Data are mean perfusion units ± SE (shown as error bar). *p<0.05 O vs I within gp at time point (reprinted with permission from Rink CL et al. [33]).*

and can vary in size and magnitude requiring prolonged recovery time out of the prosthesis, a new socket fitting and sometimes surgical interventions [26, 27].

3.3 Preserving residual limb health

Skin ulcers are typically the end result of vascular insufficiency and improper skin barrier function. Reperfusion of blood, as seen in reactive hyperemia, to nutrient- and oxygen-deprived tissue is another causative factor of tissue injury that contributes to ulcer formation [28]. In lower-limb amputation, this was identified

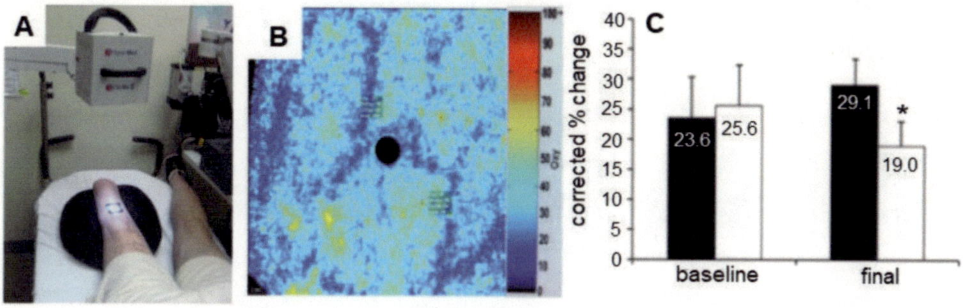

Figure 5.
*Hyperspectral imaging for skin oxygen saturation. (A) Black box represents field of view (FOV) for qualification of tissue oxygen saturation (StO_2) in residual limb. (B) Representative oxygen saturation map. (C) Reactive hyperemia quantified as percent changed in tissue oxygen saturation pre- and postactivity was determined in standard of care (SoC) (black bar) and EVS (white bar) socket systems at baseline and after 16 weeks of use (final). Data are mean ± SE (shown in error bar), *p < 0.05 SoC vs. EVS (reprinted with permission from Rink et al. [33]).*

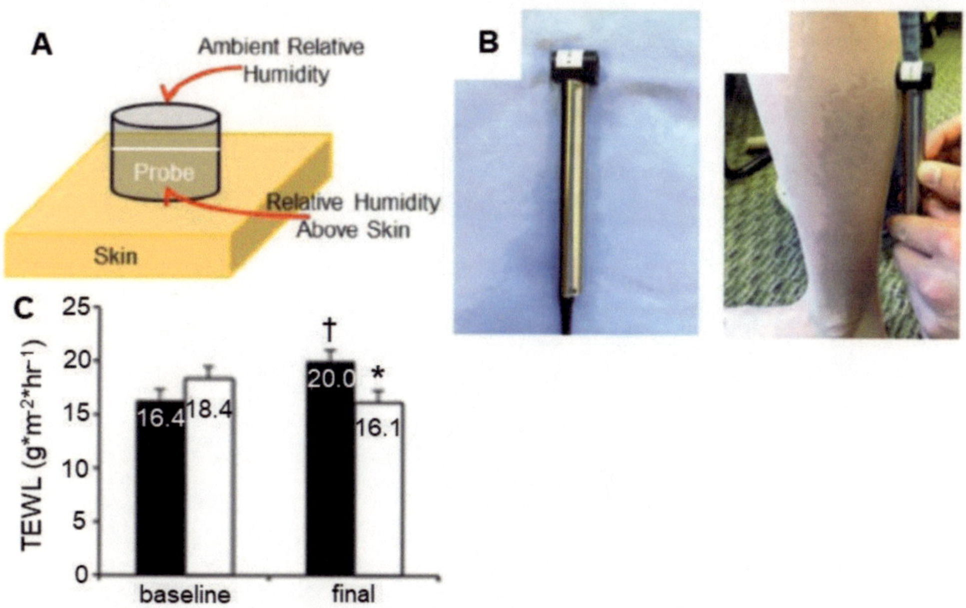

Figure 6.
*Transepidermal water loss (TEWL) for skin barrier function. (A) Schematic of TEWL probe over the skin as it measures differences between relative humidity of ambient air and directly above skin. (B) Photograph of a TEWL measurement. (C) TEWL was measured 15 min after socket doffing in people with transtibial and transfemoral amputation (n = 10) under standard of care (SoC) (black bar) and EVS (white bar) conditions. Data shown are from areas of high stress and low stress combined. Data shown are from areas of high stress and low stress combined. Data are mean ± SE (shown as error bars). *p < 0.05 SoC vs. EVS within time point. †p<0.05 baseline vs. final within prosthesis group (reprinted with permission from Rink et al. [33]).*

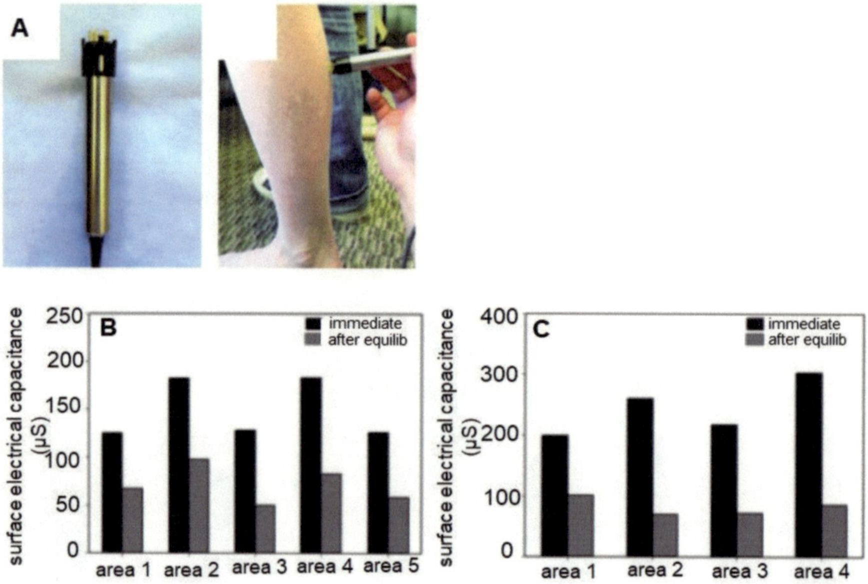

Figure 7.
Surface electrical capacitance for skin hydration. (A) Close-up view of SEC probe. Photograph of SEC measurement collection from a subject. SEC measurements from (B) transtibial and (C) transfermoral subjects immediately after liner removal and after equilibration with air for 15 min (reprinted with permission from Rink et al. [33]).

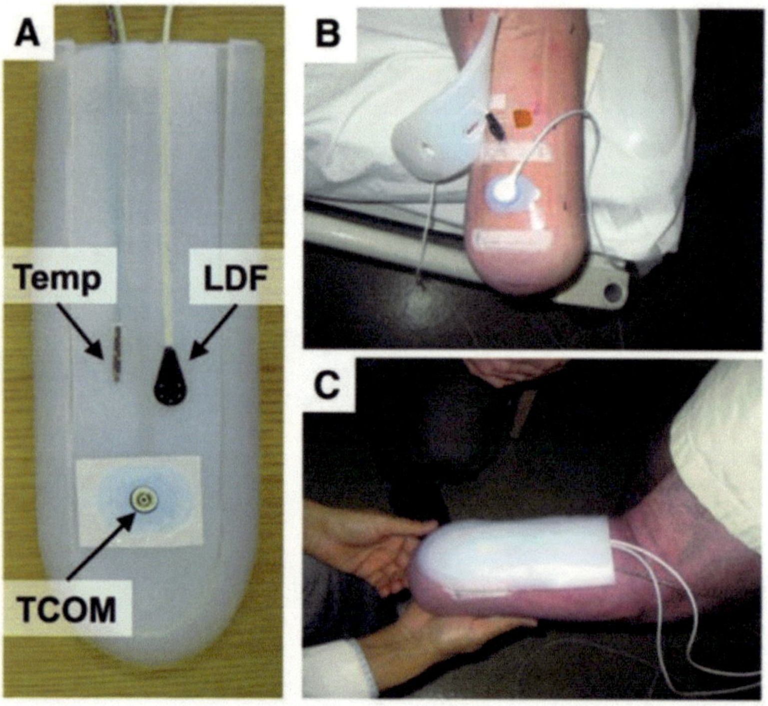

Figure 8.
Silicone gel probe holder for in-liner measurement. (A) Temperature, transcutaneous oxygen measurement (TCOM) wand laser Doppler flowmetry (LDF) probes were embedded in a silicone gel insert to enable real-time measurement of limb temperature, oxygenation, and perfusion respectively. (B) Placement of probes on residual limb of transtibial participant. Oxygen permeable Tegaderm™ was used to adhere the TCOM probe to the limb. (C) The silicone gel insert enabled reproducible placement and spacing of probes and buffered against the liner from pressing probes tightly against skin (reprinted with permission from Rink et al. [33]).

as a complication of prosthesis use in the early 1960s [29]. Key among the factors to monitor in attempting to preserve and promote residual limb health would be maintenance of skin barrier function, perfusion and oxygenation.

There are few examples of evidence based research related to the effect of socket systems, particularly elevated vacuum suspension systems on limb health [30–32]. A recent study was the first to directly test the effect of EVS on residual-limb skin health and blood flow [20]. This study used a standardized non-invasive imaging (**Figures 4**-7) approach with a combination of out-of-socket imaging (e.g., hyperspectral imaging, transepidermal water loss (TEWL) and surface electrical capacitance (SEC)) and in-socket imaging (e.g., transcutaneous oximetry (TCOM), laser Doppler flowmetry (LDF)) [20, 33]. Outcomes of this study identified that elevated vacuum suspension socket systems promote better residual limb skin physiology by preserving the skin barrier function (TEWL measurements), rescuing against loss of tissue oxygenation during activity and attenuating reactive hyperemia. Customized test sockets for people with TT and TF amputations with embedded in-socket silicone probe holder (**Figures 3** and **8**) housed perfusion (LDF) and tissue oxygen (TCOM) measurement probes and enabled multiple temporal measurements from the same sites to be taken in study without the individual probes interfering with one another.

4. Summary and conclusions

Residual limb skin health is a key determinant of quality of life for individuals with lower limb amputation. Skin health problems, caused by shear forces and stress to the residual limb, are known to affect the ability of individuals with lower limb loss to perform household tasks, use their prosthesis, engage in social functions, and participate in sports. Therefore, objective measures to during socket fitting combined with real-time monitoring of skin physiological parameters such as barrier function, hydration and perfusion are likely to provide a better fitting and functional artificial limb for long-term use.

Acknowledgements

The authors acknowledge grant funding from the United States Department of Defense (DoD) Congressionally Directed Medical Research Programs (CDMRP) grant award W81XWH-16-2-0059.

Conflict of interest

The authors declare no conflict of interest.

Author details

Sashwati Roy, Shomita S. Mathew-Steiner and Chandan K. Sen*
Indiana University School of Medicine, Indianapolis, IN, USA

*Address all correspondence to: cksen@iu.edu

References

[1] Lake C. The evolution of upper limb prosthetic socket design. Journal of Prosthetics and Orthotics. 2008;**20**:85

[2] Schultz AE, Baade SP, Kuiken TA. Expert opinions on success factors for upper-limb prostheses. Journal of Rehabilitation Research and Development. 2007;**44**(4):483-489

[3] Berke G. Post-operative management of the lower extremity amputee: Standards of care. Official findings of the state-of-the-science conferences #2. Journal of Prosthetics and Orthotics. 2004;**16**:6-12

[4] Zachariah SG, Saxena R, Fergason JR, Sanders JE. Shape and volume change in the transtibial residuum over the short term: Preliminary investigation of six subjects. Journal of Rehabilitation Research and Development. 2004;**41**(5):683-694

[5] Fernie GR, Holliday PJ. Volume fluctuations in the residual limbs of lower limb amputees. Archives of Physical Medicine and Rehabilitation. 1982;**63**(4):162-165

[6] Sanders JE, Fatone S. Residual limb volume change: Systematic review of measurement and management. Journal of Rehabilitation Research and Development. 2011;**48**(8):949-986

[7] Turney BW, Kent SJ, Walker RT, Loftus IM. Amputations: No longer the end of the road. Journal of the Royal College of Surgeons of Edinburgh. 2001;**46**(5):271-273

[8] Taylor SM, Kalbaugh CA, Blackhurst DW, Hamontree SE, Cull DL, Messich HS, et al. Preoperative clinical factors predict postoperative functional outcomes after major lower limb amputation: An analysis of 553 consecutive patients. Journal of Vascular Surgery. 2005;**42**(2):227-235

[9] Ziegler-Graham K, MacKenzie EJ, Ephraim PL, Travison TG, Brookmeyer R. Estimating the prevalence of limb loss in the United States: 2005 to 2050. Archives of Physical Medicine and Rehabilitation. 2008;**89**(3):422-429

[10] Epstein RA, Heinemann AW, McFarland LV. Quality of life for veterans and servicemembers with major traumatic limb loss from Vietnam and OIF/OEF conflicts. Journal of Rehabilitation Research and Development. 2010;**47**(4):373-385

[11] Krueger CA, Wenke JC, Ficke JR. Ten years at war: Comprehensive analysis of amputation trends. Journal of Trauma and Acute Care Surgery. 2012;**73**(6 Suppl 5):S438-S444

[12] Ramasamy A, Hill AM, Phillip R, Gibb I, Bull AM, Clasper JC. The modern "deck-slap" injury—Calcaneal blast fractures from vehicle explosions. The Journal of Trauma. 2011;**71**(6):1694-1698

[13] Bui KM, Raugi GJ, Nguyen VQ, Reiber GE. Skin problems in individuals with lower-limb loss: Literature review and proposed classification system. Journal of Rehabilitation Research and Development. 2009;**46**(9):1085-1090

[14] Harris AM, Althausen PL, Kellam J, Bosse MJ, Castillo R. Lower extremity assessment project study G. Complications following limb-threatening lower extremity trauma. Journal of Orthopaedic Trauma. 2009;**23**(1):1-6

[15] Klute GK, Kantor C, Darrouzet C, Wild H, Wilkinson S, Iveljic S, et al. Lower-limb amputee needs assessment using multistakeholder focus-group approach. Journal of Rehabilitation Research and Development. 2009;**46**(3):293-304

[16] Pezzin LE, Dillingham TR, Mackenzie EJ, Ephraim P, Rossbach P. Use and satisfaction with prosthetic limb devices and related services. Archives of Physical Medicine and Rehabilitation. 2004;**85**(5):723-729

[17] Legro MW, Reiber G, del Aguila M, Ajax MJ, Boone DA, Larsen JA, et al. Issues of importance reported by persons with lower limb amputations and prostheses. Journal of Rehabilitation Research and Development. 1999;**36**(3):155-163

[18] Convery P, Murray KD. Ultrasound study of the motion of the residual femur within a trans-femoral socket during gait. Prosthetics and Orthotics International. 2000;**24**(3):226-232

[19] Sanders JE, Karchin A, Fergason JR, Sorenson EA. A noncontact sensor for measurement of distal residual-limb position during walking. Journal of Rehabilitation Research and Development. 2006;**43**(4):509-516

[20] Rink C, Wernke MM, Powell HM, Gynawali S, Schroeder RM, Kim JY, et al. Elevated vacuum suspension preserves residual-limb skin health in people with lower-limb amputation: Randomized clinical trial. JRRD is now PLOS Veterans Disability & Rehabilitation Research Channel. California: PLOS; 2016;**53**(6):1121-1132

[21] Wernke MM, Schroeder RM, Haynes ML, Nolt LL, Albury AW, Colvin JM. Progress toward optimizing prosthetic socket fit and suspension using elevated vacuum to promote residual limb health. Advances in Wound Care. 2017;**6**(7):233-239

[22] Hoskins RD, Sutton EE, Kinor D, Schaeffer JM, Fatone S. Using vacuum-assisted suspension to manage residual limb wounds in persons with transtibial amputation: A case series. Prosthetics and Orthotics International. 2014;**38**(1):68-74

[23] Sanders JE, Zachariah SG, Jacobsen AK, Fergason JR. Changes in interface pressures and shear stresses over time on trans-tibial amputee subjects ambulating with prosthetic limbs: Comparison of diurnal and six-month differences. Journal of Biomechanics. 2005;**38**(8):1566-1573

[24] Meulenbelt HE, Geertzen JH, Jonkman MF, Dijkstra PU. Skin problems of the stump in lower limb amputees: 1. A clinical study. Acta Dermato-Venereologica. 2011;**91**(2):173-177

[25] Hagberg K, Branemark R. Consequences of non-vascular trans-femoral amputation: A survey of quality of life, prosthetic use and problems. Prosthetics and Orthotics International. 2001;**25**(3):186-194

[26] Highsmith JT, Highsmith MJ. Common skin pathology in LE prosthesis users. JAAPA: Official Journal of the American Academy of Physician Assistants. 2007;**20**(11):33, 47-36

[27] Highsmith MJ, Kahle JT, Klenow TD, Andrews CR, Lewis KL, Bradley RC, et al. Interventions to manage residual limb ulceration due to prosthetic use IN individuals with lower extremity amputation: A systematic review of the literature. Technology and Innovation. 2016;**18**(2-3):115-123

[28] Peirce SM, Skalak TC, Rodeheaver GT. Ischemia-reperfusion injury in chronic pressure ulcer formation: A skin model in the rat. Wound Repair and Regeneration. 2000;**8**(1):68-76

[29] Levy SW, Allende MF, Barnes GH. Skin problems of the leg amputee. Archives of Dermatology. 1962;**85**:65-81

[30] Kahle JTOJ, Johnston W, Highsmith JM. The effects of vacuum-assisted suspension on residual limb physiology, wound healing and function: A systematic review. Technology and Innovation. 2014;**15**:333-341

[31] Kahle JT, Highsmith MJ. Transfemoral sockets with vacuum-assisted suspension comparison of hip kinematics, socket position, contact pressure, and preference: Ischial containment versus brimless. Journal of Rehabilitation Research and Development. 2013;**50**(9):1241-1252

[32] Board WJ, Street GM, Caspers C. A comparison of trans-tibial amputee suction and vacuum socket conditions. Prosthetics and Orthotics International. 2001;**25**(3):202-209

[33] Rink CL, Wernke MM, Powell HM, Tornero M, Gnyawali SC, Schroeder RM, et al. Standardized approach to quantitatively measure residual limb skin health in individuals with lower limb amputation. Advances in Wound Care. New York: Mary Ann Liebert; 2017;**6**(7):225-232

Chapter 5

Ambulatory Devices: Assessment and Prescription

Daniel Olufemi Odebiyi and Caleb Adewumi Adeagbo

Abstract

Injuries or disabilities associated with the lower extremities and aging frequently result in ambulation difficulty and this usually necessitates the prescription of ambulatory assistive device (e.g., cane, crutch and walker) in an attempt to restore locomotory function. Ambulatory devices are orthotic devices that provide support, stability and balance for users to able to move from one point to another. Users can progress or retrogress from one ambulatory device to another while some are permanently fit on a particular device throughout lifetime. The progression is dependent on the medical condition, user's abilities, user's anthropometric and environment. Physiotherapist prescribes ambulatory device to users and helps with the fitting and proper use of the ambulatory device. A correct prescription and well fitted ambulatory device minimize functional limitation and promote functional ability and improve quality of life. Incorrect prescription, fitting and use of ambulatory device may result in early fatigue, frustration, fall and damage to blood vessels, muscles or nerves.

Keywords: ambulatory devices, walker, crutches, cane

1. Introduction

Ambulatory devices are mobility devices that assist in transfer of user from one point to another. Ambulatory devices require active participation of users during mobilization while mobility devices requires passive participation of users. Mobility devices are stretchers and wheelchairs [37].

Ambulatory devices are used by people with musculoskeletal impairments, neurological deficit and older people in order to be independent or decrease dependency on care-givers and health care practitioners. Ambulatory devices are orthotic devices used for support (i.e., augmentation of muscle action and/or reduction of weight-bearing load), maintaining stability and balance with the aim of transferring individual with ambulatory difficulty from one point to another due to injury or disability [13].

Many factors predispose an individual to use ambulatory devices. These factors may be aging, congenital, medical or traumatic. Congenital factors include structural deformities that are present at birth, while traumatic factors are as a result of accident. Medical factors are as a result of diseases which can lead to amputation, limb discrepancies, muscle weakness and loss of balance. Users can progress or retrogress from one ambulatory device to another while some are permanently fit on a particular device throughout lifetime.

There are many ambulatory devices developed to suit diverse presentations from difference medical or surgical conditions and these include parallel bar, walker, crutches and cane. Each of the ambulatory device has advantages and disadvantages that enhance their prescription and usage. Therefore, clinicians need to have a good understanding of these ambulatory devices to be able to recommend the ideal ambulatory device for the user [3, 10].

Prescription of ambulatory device is determined by the user's anthropometric parameters (body weight, height and body mass index), user's abilities (skill), user's needs and environment. Other factors that influence the prescription of ambulatory devices include; weight bearing status, the degree of support or assistance the device can offer, the coordination of the user, range of motion available at the involved joints, balance, stability, strength, and general condition of the user.

There are also body functions involved in determining user's capacity to use an ambulatory device, these are cognitive function, judgment, vision, vestibular function, upper body strength, physical endurance. Depending on severity, impairments in any of these functions could make it impossible for a user to safely use a device.

The prescription of any ambulatory device should specify the device most likely to maximize the user's function; the individual's goals and personal preferences must also be considered. Physiotherapists are licensed and help with the fitting and proper use of ambulatory device while other health practitioners can also recommend ambulatory devices. All ambulatory devices are made in different height and so user must be fitted in order to obtain the correct ambulatory device height [6].

The functions of ambulatory devices when properly use includes the following:

- Provides assist forward, backward and lateral movements: users of an ambulatory device can walk in any direction with and within the device.

- Helps to increase balance, stability and coordination of the users: there is increase balance due to the increase in the base of support provided by the ambulatory devices (**Figure 1**).

- Helps to reduce weight bearing on the affected lower limb: use of ambulatory devices result in the upper limbs sharing weight bearing with the affected lower limbs, thereby reducing the weight of the body of user being borne on the affected lower limbs.

- Helps to increase confidence of the users: the user can move independently without or with little manual assistance.

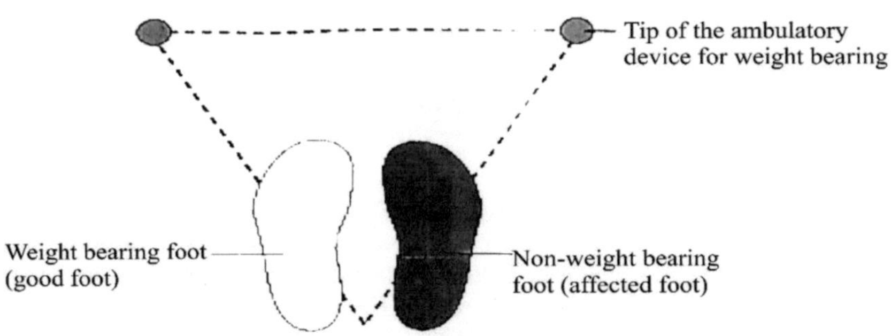

Figure 1.
Increase of the base of support for a user of ambulatory device (crutches).

- Helps to correct poor posture: the support provided by ambulatory devices creates a platform that enhances good posture habit among users when the right ambulatory device is selected and properly fit.

- Helps to reduce risk of fall: assumption of good posture arising from increased supporting base of users help to reduce the risk of fall among users.

- Helps to reduce pain on the affected limb: the use of ambulatory support encourages body weight of the users to transferred to the ambulatory devices.

- Helps to augment muscular strength of the trunk and of the affected lower limbs [21].

2. Ambulatory devices

Ambulatory devices are aids made of durable and non-malleable materials for assistance during walking and standing. The main function of ambulatory device is to reduce the amount of weight bearing on the weak (or affected) lower limb or totally eliminate weight from the lower limb by transmitting the body weight from the upper limb to the floor through the ambulatory device [8]. Weight bearing status of ambulatory device user is the amount of weight the user put on the weak (or affected) lower limb during ambulation. The weight bearing status can be measured in grades or percentages. The amount of weight bearing on the weak (or affected) lower limb is determined by the user medical history, weight bearing capacity as can be tolerated and functional ability of the weak (or affected) lower limb [11]. The weight bearing status available among ambulatory device users (apart from cane) are as described below:

Non-weight bearing (*NWB*): the affected lower limb will not touch the floor during ambulation (i.e., no weight is borne on the affected lower limb) [11]. The percentage of body weight transmitted to the floor, through the affected lower limb is zero (0)% (**Figure 2**).

Touch down weight bearing (*TDWB*): this is also known as toe touch weight bearing (TTWB). Here, the foot or the toes touch the floor but no weight is transmitted to the floor through the affected lower limb involved. Thus, the percentage of body weight transmitted to the floor, through the affected lower limb is also zero (0)% (**Figure 3**).

Partial weight bearing (*PWB*): here, a little amount of weight is transmitted to the floor through the affected lower limb. The percentage of body weight transmitted to the floor can range between 1 and 50% [11]. During the training stage, two body weighing machines/apparatus can be used to accurately determine the percentage body that may borne on the affected lower limb (**Figure 4**).

Weight bearing as tolerated (*WBT*): the user of the ambulatory device determines the amount of weight to bear on the affected/involved lower limb. The weight bearing status is totally dependent on the individual ambulatory device user and the percentage of body weight transmitted to the floor can range from 50 to 100% [11].

Full weight bearing (*FWB*): the affected/involved lower limb can bear the total weight of the body. The percentage of body weight transmitted to the floor through the affected lower limb can be 100% [11]. This type of weight bearing status is used to build confidence with the ambulatory device user.

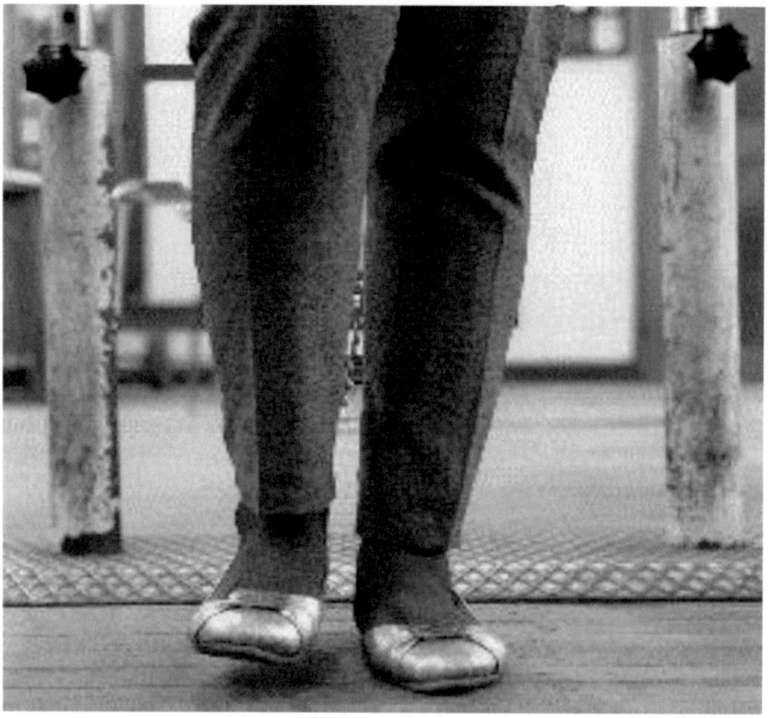

Figure 2.
Non-weight bearing (NWB) on the right lower limb. The non-weight bearing limb is not touching the floor.

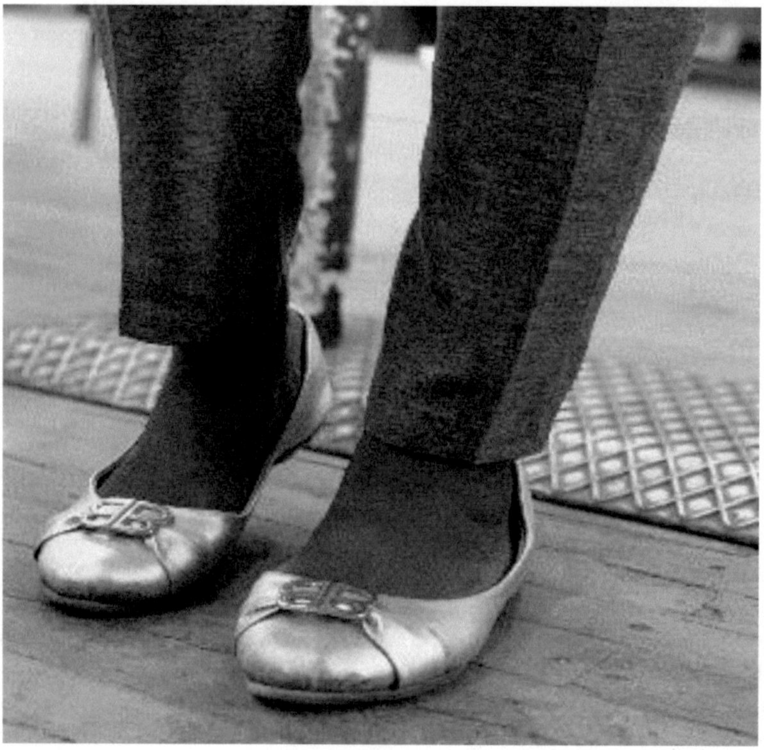

Figure 3.
Touch down weight bearing (TDWB) on the right lower limb. The reference lower limb is only touching the floor but not bearing weight.

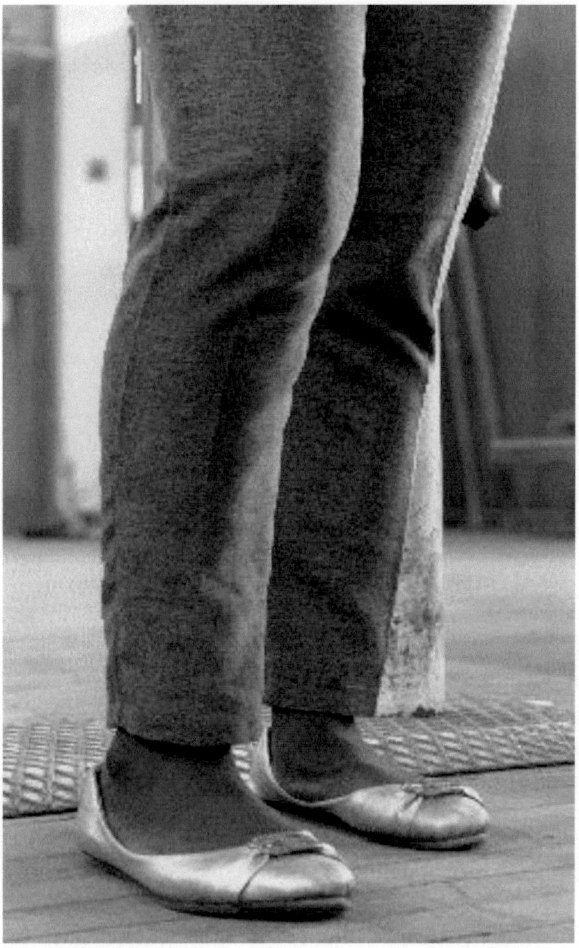

Figure 4.
Partial weight bearing (PWB) or weight bearing as tolerated (WBT) on the right lower limb. The weight the reference lower limb bear is decided by the amount of weight that can be tolerated.

3. Categories of ambulatory device

Ambulatory devices can be group into categories depending on the basic design. When arranged in the level of stability of the ambulatory device the progression is parallel bar, walker, crutches and cane. Each of the categories of the ambulatory device is then redesign and modify to different styles and types to specifically meet the needs of the user.

4. Parallel bar

4.1 Description and components of parallel bar

Parallel bar are fixed apparatus with a pair of horizontal bars on vertical posts used for standing and ambulatory training (**Figure 5**). It is a medical ambulatory device with two parallel horizontal bars on fixed four legs; the user holds the horizontal bars at wrist height and move forward, backward and sideways, usually

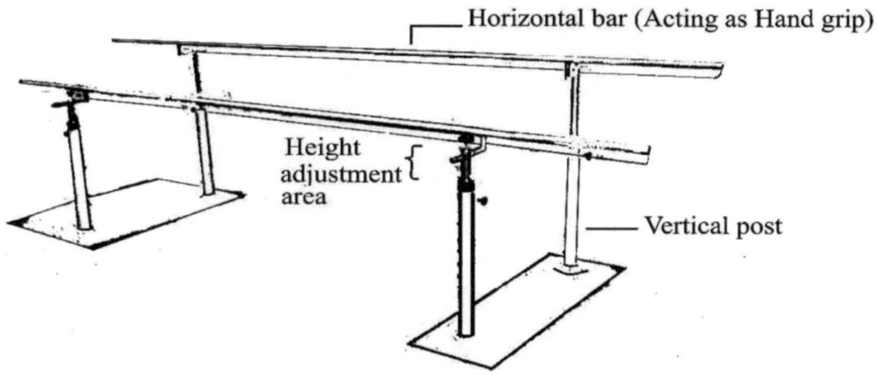

Figure 5.
Parallel bar fixed together for stability. There are knobs on the vertical poles for adjusting the height.

in front of a standing mirror. Each of the horizontal bars is mounted on two adjustable vertical posts to allow for easy adjustment of height of the parallel in accordance with the anthropometric parameters of the users. The entire horizontal bars form the handgrip for the users. The vertical posts are fixed to the floor or joined together for stability of the parallel bar. The horizontal bars are about 18 inches apart; and are set at the same height by the vertical posts which are about 11 feet (340 cm) long. Pediatric parallel bars are also available with adjustable height. The horizontal bars are usually made of wood; while the vertical posts are made of different materials such as stainless steel, aluminum steel or iron. The material used to manufacture the parallel bar determines the weight, durability, cost, strength, comfort and safety.

4.2 Advantages of parallel bar

1. It provides maximum stability: the fact that users (patients) are positioned between the two parallel bars gives room for further stability in addition to the presence of the therapists at either side of users.

2. It requires the least amount of coordination: the present of the two parallel bars also makes coordination a lot easier; as users holds onto the bars as he/she moves along.

3. It is the best ambulatory device to practice ambulation, particularly at the onset of ambulatory training. As it creates confidence in the patient and also reduce the fear of falling in the patient.

4. It can be used to determine other ambulatory device the user will use because the patient performance within the parallel bar will indicate the ability to use other type of ambulatory devices.

4.3 Disadvantages of parallel bar

1. User's ambulation is limited within and between the parallel bar, although guided by the mirror positioned at the other end of the parallel bars.

2. It is stationary (usually not moveable): parallel bars are usually permanently positioned at a particular place in the treatment room or medical gymnasium. The patient has to be moved (usually on wheelchair) to the parallel bars.

3. It is expensive compared to other ambulatory devices: it is not readily made available for home use because the financial implication involved in building it. Thus, its usage usually requires moving the patient (users) to the facility (i.e., hospital).

4.4 Fitting of parallel bar

Parallel bars are usually adjustable, the heights of the bars are adjusted to fit the user. The adjustment is estimated base on the user's height. The bars should be at the level of the greater trochanter of the user and the elbow joint should be able to flex to about 20 or 30 degrees when the user grips the horizontal bars. Further adjustment of the heights of the bars is made, with the view to fit the parallel bars to the user's height, immediately the user is position in standing position, where there is need. Usually the adjustment of the parallel bar is fixed at two- and half-inch interval or less depending on the manufacturer and the user (adult or pediatric).

4.5 Instruction on the use of parallel bar

Prior to ambulation using the parallel bar, the following safety and precautions should be checked.

- The stability of the parallel bar should be checked. All the vertical posts (limbs) of the parallel bar should be fixed, stabilized and immovable.
- All the push buttons for height adjustment should be visible and at the same height level.
- The handgrips on the horizontal bars should be attached sturdily and not move when pressure applied.
- There should be no loose component (screw, nuts or bolt) in the parallel bar.
- No dents, cracks or any irregularities on the parallel bar.

Also, the following instructions should be given to the users before they are positioned between the parallel bars:

- Users should maintain good posture (hyper flexion of the head, neck and trunk should be avoided).
- Users should hold the horizontal bars firmly.

Users of parallel bars first need to learn how to stand using the parallel bar. The user uses one of the upper limbs to hold one bars of the parallel bar (for stability and balance) and the other upper limb to assist in standing by pushing up on the seat (**Figure 6A**). Clinicians can assist the user into standing position from sitting by assisting the user from the axilla region. Immediately the user is almost standing user change the position of the upper limb that was on the seat to the other bar of the parallel bars (**Figure 6B**). User stands upright within the walker, adjusting the upper limb and lower limb till the user is balance.

When siting from standing using the parallel bar, the user follow the reverse pattern of standing. From upright standing within the parallel bar, the user place

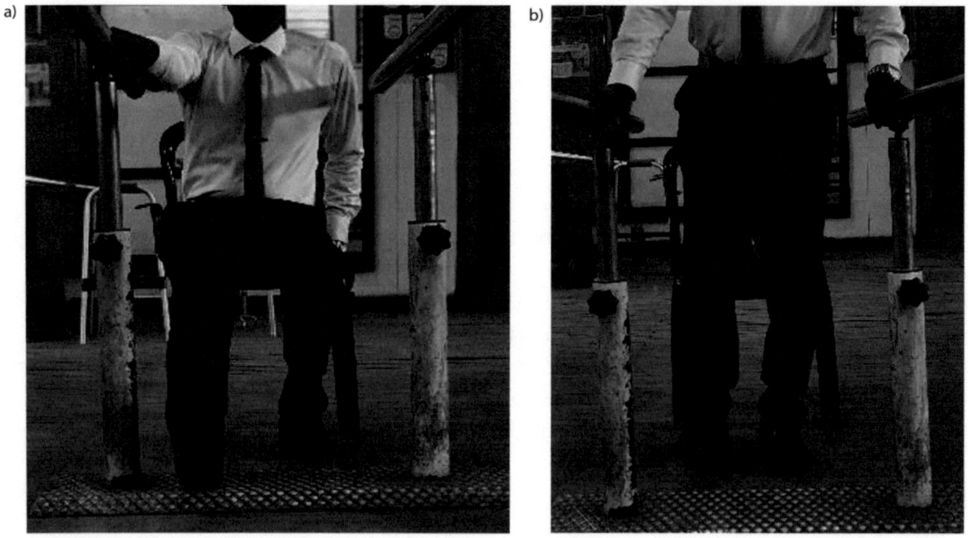

Figure 6.
Positioning for learning how to use the parallel bars: (a) learning how to stand when using the parallel bar, (b) moving the hand on the seat to the horizontal pole of the parallel bar to maintain stability.

one hand (i.e., upper limb) on the seat to control the speed and bear weight of sitting. Then the user sits gradually, using the other upper limb on the bar to control the movement back to seating.

4.6 Weight bearing status possible with parallel bar

The following weight bearing status can be used with parallel bar: non-weight bearing (NWB), touch down weight bearing (TDWB), partial weight bearing (PWB), weight bearing as tolerated (WBT), full weight bearing (FWB).

4.7 Non-weight bearing (NWB)

The user slides the upper limbs on the horizontal bars forward to an arm's length (weight of the body is on unaffected lower limb and the affected lower limb is not touching the ground). The user shared his/her body weight between the unaffected lower limb and parallel bar by putting body weight on the parallel bar using the upper limbs. The user then moves the affects/involved lower limb (freely without bearing weight, i.e., NWB) forward and finally moves his/her body (weight), by propelling himself/herself forward (hopping) using the upper limbs to complete the cycle. The user is made to repeat this cycle in order to continue to move forward.

4.8 Touch-down weight bearing (TDWB)

The user slides the upper limbs on the horizontal bars forward to an arm's length distance, with the body weight borne on unaffected lower limb while allowing the foot or toes of the affected lower limb to touch the ground without bearing any weight. Then the user put body weight on the parallel bar using the upper limbs and moves himself/herself forward, completing the cycle. This way the user finally moves forward. The user is made to repeat this cycle in order to continue to move forward.

4.9 Partial weight bearing (PWB)

The user slides the upper limbs on the horizontal bars forward to an arm's length distance. Then the user puts weight on the parallel bar using the upper limbs and moves the affected/involved lower limb forward (bearing less than 50% of body weight on the affected/involved lower limb). And the other 50% body weight is shared between unaffected lower limb and the horizontal bars. The user finally moves forward to complete the cycle. The user is made to repeat this cycle in order to continue to move forward.

4.10 Weight bearing as tolerated (WBT)

While standing and sharing the body weight on the unaffected lower limb and the horizontal bars, the user slides the upper limbs on the horizontal bars forward to an arm's length distance. Then the user moves forward by taking the affected/involved lower limb forward, bearing body weight that the lower limb can tolerate on the affected/involved lower limb, and finally moves the weight bearing lower limb. This cycle is then repeated. User can learn normal walking by putting one leg ahead of the other during ambulation.

4.11 Full weight bearing (FWB)

The user slides the upper limbs on the horizontal bars forward to an arm's length distance. Then the user hold the parallel bar using the upper limbs and moves the affected/involved lower limb forward (bearing full body weight on the lower limb) and finally moves the weight bearing lower limb forward (same or different level as the FWB lower limb). Then cycle is then repeated.

5. Walker

5.1 Description and components

Walker is also known as walking frame or called zimmer frame. It is a modified and mobile version of the parallel bar (**Figure 7**). It is a medical ambulatory device

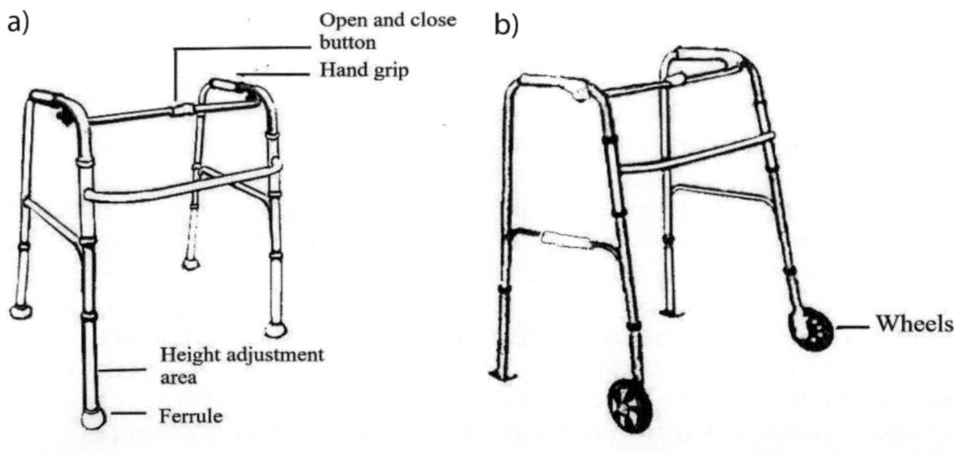

Figure 7.
Two types of walkers (walking frame); (a) with four rubber ferrules and (b) two rubber ferrules behind and two wheel rollers in front.

with about four legs or less in which the user holds the handle bars at wrist height and place the device in front during movement (**Figure** 7). It has horizontal bars on vertical posts for adjustment and folding. It has a permanent hand grip and rubber ferrules. The horizontal bars are about 18 inches apart to fit the body of the user while the height can be adjusted by the vertical posts. Adult walker height is between 32 and 37 inches (81–92 cm). Pediatric walkers are also available with adjustable height [16].

The parts that formed the walker include handgrip, ferrule (or wheels), open and close button (for folding or collapsing the walker), push buttons (for adjustment of the height of the walker). The horizontal bars and vertical posts are made of different materials such as wood, hard plastic, stainless steel, aluminum steel and iron. The material used to manufacture the walker determines the weight, durability, cost, strength, comfort and safety.

5.2 Advantages of walker

1. It is good for users with poor balance and coordination.

2. It can be used to decrease weight bearing to both lower extremities.

3. It is the best to prescribe to the elderly.

4. It is the best to prescribe to the obese.

5. It is the best to prescribe to for long distance without getting fatigue in user that lack endurance.

6. It can be used to train endurance.

5.3 Disadvantages of walker

1. It cannot be used in crowded environment or cluttered setting.

2. It cannot be used for stair climbing.

3. It is not appropriate for rough terrain.

5.4 Types of walkers

Standard walker: has four legs with ferrule (no mobile base) (**Figure** 7**A**). The user requires strength and grip power to lift the entire frame forward during ambulation.

Wheeled walker: the design is similar to the standard walker but the ferrules are replaced by wheels (**Figure 7B**). The number of wheels depends on the strength and stability of the user. The user only needs strength tilt the ambulatory device move forward. The wheeled walker can be 2-wheeled walker or 4-wheeled walker. Some design can come in with three legs instead of four and the three legs will be wheeled. Some walkers are design with hand brake for stability. The wheeled walker is better than the standard walker because the user require less energy to move the device forward. However, it is better prescribed for stable users, who can control the walker reasonably. Another disadvantage of 2-wheeled and standard walker is that they cannot be swivel by user when turning, they need to be carried but the 4-wheeled walker and 3-wheeled walker can be swivel. There are two different folding styles for walkers. The folding help for easy transportation and storage of the device

1. Hinged front legs: the folding mechanism is activated by pulling a ball mounted on a piece of string. When the ball is pulled towards the user, the brace bar situated around the bottom of the frame slides up. At the same time the front section moves inwards until the front and back legs meet. This mechanism offers the user the choice of reducing the size of the walker.

2. Side folding frame: the locking motion on the walker is activated by the user pressing on the close and open button on the front horizontal bar of the frame. This therefore allows each side to be folded in to meet the front section. Once fully retracted, this type of frame becomes completely flat and more space efficient.

Other forms of walkers are:

Forearm walker: this type of walker is basically the same as the standard walking frame but with forearm support rather than handgrips. This allows the user to transfer their weight through their forearms rather than their hands. This is particularly helpful to those who have arthritic hands and find gripping the frame challenging.

Reciprocal walker: a reciprocal walker operates with a pivot mechanism for each side. This provides the user with the option of lifting the frame up and moving around one step at a time. Many users prefer this movement as it is more intuitive to how one naturally walks. However, consideration needs to be given to how much weight is being placed on one side of the body, specifically arms. It is advisable to consult a physiotherapist or other health practitioner about the suitability of this frame.

5.5 Fitting a walker

Walkers are usually adjustable; the height of the walker is adjusted to fit the user. The adjustment is estimated base on the user's height. The height of the walker should be at the level of the greater trochanter of the user and the elbow joint should be able to flex to about 20 or 30 degrees when user hold the hand grip of the frame in an upright position. Immediately the user stand and the horizontal bars are too short or too tall for the user the user is allow to sit and the horizontal bars are adjusted to fit the user height.

5.6 Safety and precautionary measures when using a walker

Prior to ambulation using a walker, the following safety and precautions should be checked.

- The stability of the walker should be checked. All the vertical posts (limbs) of the walker should touch the floor.

- The open and close button should be in open position.

- All the push button should be visible and same level.

- The ferrules or wheels are not loose or worn out.

- The handgrips are attached sturdily and not move when pressure is applied.
- No component should be found loosen in the walker.
- There should be no dents, cracks or any irregularities on the walker.

5.7 Instruction on how to use a walker

The following instructions should be given to the user before use:

- User should maintain good posture (hyper flexion of the head, neck and trunk should be avoided).
- User should avoid moving too close to the front horizontal bars.
- User should avoid staying too far away from the walker.
- Users should not use walker for stair climbing.

5.8 Weight bearing status used with walkers

The following weight bearing status can be used with walkers: non-weight bearing (NWB), touch down weight bearing (TDWB), partial weight bearing (PWB), weight bearing as tolerated (WBT), full weight bearing (FWB).

The user first need to learn how to stand using the walker. The user uses one of the upper limb to hold the walker (for stability and balance) and the other upper limb to assist in standing (pushing on the seat). Clinicians can assist the user into standing position from sitting by assisting the user from the axilla region. Immediately the user is almost standing user change the position of the upper limb that was on the seat to the walker. User stands upright within the walker, adjusting the upper limb and lower limb till the user is balance. User will sit by following the opposite procedure of standing. User first make sure the lower limbs are touching the seat then use one upper limb to hold the seat and user gradually sit on the seat and remove the other upper limb to adjust the position on the chair.

5.9 Non-weight bearing (NWB)

The user moves the walker forward to about an arm's length distance, with the weight of the body is on the unaffected/involved lower limb (i.e., weight bearing lower limb) and the affected lower limb is not touching the ground. Then the user put his/her weight on the walker using the upper limbs and moves the affected/involved (i.e., NWB lower limb) forward towards the walker and finally moves the weight bearing lower limb towards the walker (to the same level as the NWB lower limb). Then cycle is then repeated.

5.10 touch down weight bearing (TDWB)

The user moves the walker forward to an arm's length distance, with weight of the body is on unaffected lower limb and the affected lower limb foot or toes is touching the ground but not bearing weight. Then the user put the weight on the walker using the upper limbs and moves the affected/involved lower limb (i.e., TDWB lower limb) forward towards the walker (the foot or toes touching the ground but not bearing weight) and finally moves the weight bearing lower limb towards the walker (to the same level as the TDWB lower limb). The cycle is then repeated.

5.11 Partial weight bearing (PWB)

The user moves the walker forward to an arm's length distance. Then the user put the weight on the walker using the upper limbs and moves the affected/involved (i.e., PWB) lower limb forward towards the walker, bearing less than 50% of body weight on the PWB lower limb and finally moves the weight bearing lower limb towards the walker (to the same level as the PWB lower limb). The cycle is then repeated.

5.12 Weight bearing as tolerated (WBT)

The user moves the walker forward to an arm's length distance. Then the user put the weight on the walker using the upper limbs and moves the affected/involved (i.e., WBT) lower limb forward towards the walker, bearing body weight that the lower limb can tolerate on the WBT lower limb. The user finally moves the weight bearing lower limb towards the walker (to the same level as the WBT lower limb). The cycle is then repeated.

5.13 Full weight bearing (FWB)

The user moves the walker forward to an arm's length distance. Then the user put the weight on the walker using the upper limbs and moves the affected/involved (i.e., FWB) lower limb forward towards the walker (bearing total of body weight on the FWB lower limb) while moving the unaffected lower limb, i.e., the weight bearing lower limb towards the walker (to the same level as the FWB lower limb). Then cycle is then repeated.

6. Crutches

Crutches are the most common prescribed ambulatory devices. They are used in pair. Crutches have two contacts with the body (hand and elbow or hand and axilla) which make it a better ambulatory device for stabilization of the user. They are types of orthosis that provide support from the floor to the upper limb. There are two different types of crutches: axillary crutch and elbow crutch [16].

Axillary crutch: this is also known as the standard crutch. It has the following components: axillary bar covered with an axillary pad, a hand grip, and double uprights vertical posts joined distally by a single vertical post (allow height adjustment) covered with a ferrule (**Figure 8**). The adjustment of the handgrip is performed by adjusting the handgrip in predrilled holes in the double upright bars using screws and wing bolts. The vertical posts and short horizontal bars are made of different materials such as wood, hard plastic, stainless steel, aluminum steel and iron.

Adjustment of height of the axillary crutch and the handgrip is standardized in an inch distance (2.54 cm). Adult axillary crutch range from 48 to 60 inches (122–153 cm). It is available in Pediatric, youth, adult and tall adult sizes (**Figure 10** and **Table 1**).

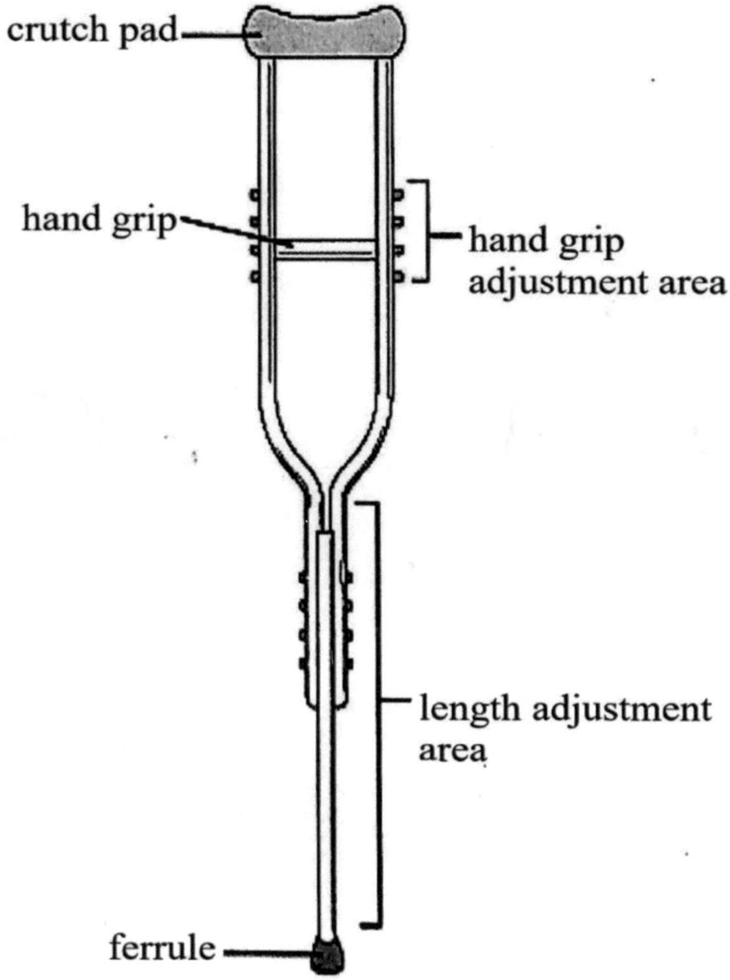

Figure 8.
Axillary crutch and its features.

6.1 Advantages

1. It is used to reduce weight bearing on one lower limb.

2. It is used to improve balance.

3. It is used to improve lateral stability.

4. It can be used for stair climbing.

6.2 Disadvantages

1. It need upper limb strength and coordination.

2. It need some trunk support.

3. It need good trunk stability.

DOI: http://dx.doi.org/10.5772/intechopen.89886

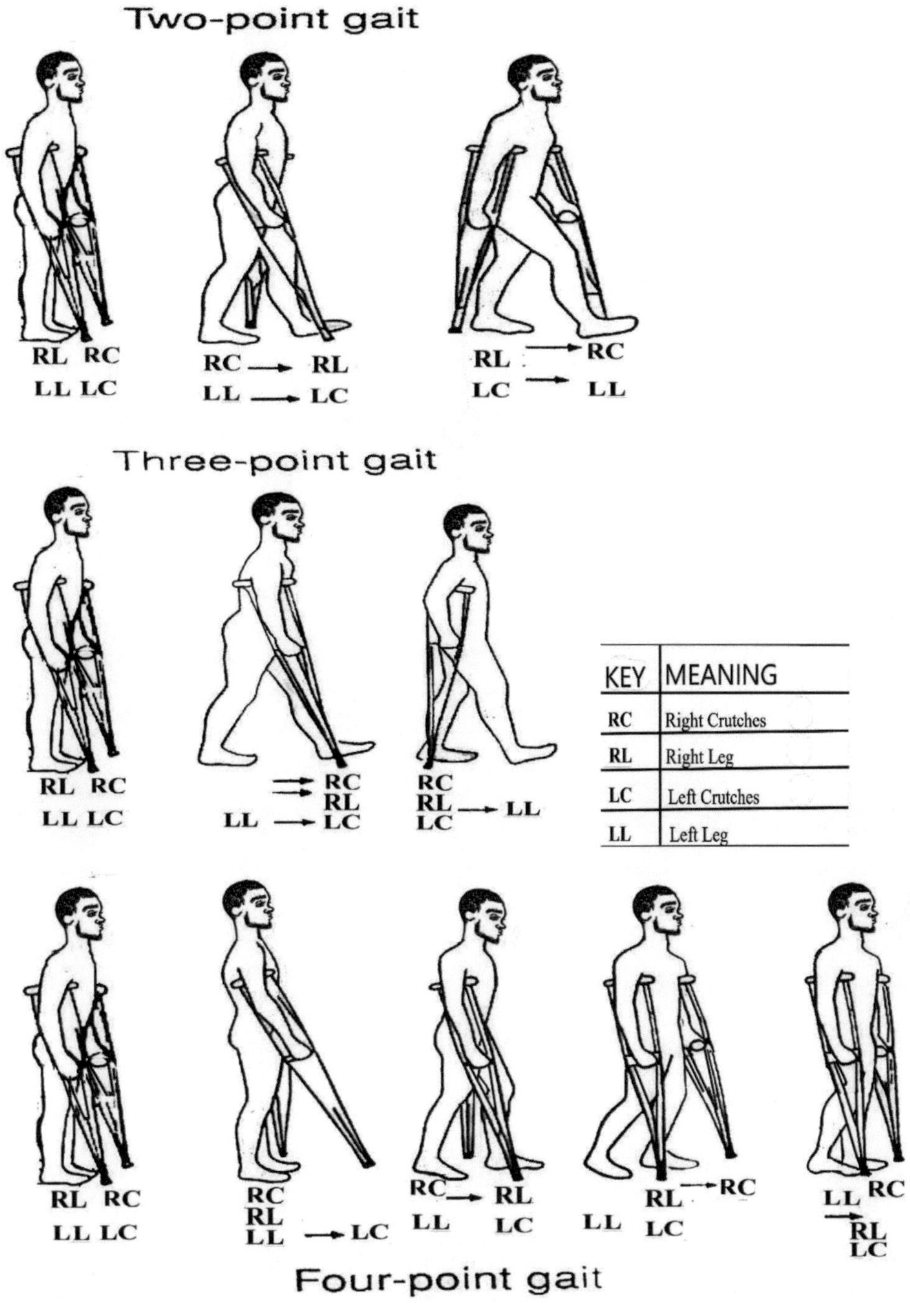

Figure 9.
Diagram of different axillary crutch walking.

6.3 Measurement for axillary crutches

There are several techniques of estimating and predicting axillary crutch length for users. The following techniques can be used: foot-head linear techniques, arm span techniques and foot-anterior axillary fold linear techniques [1, 2, 4, 5, 32].

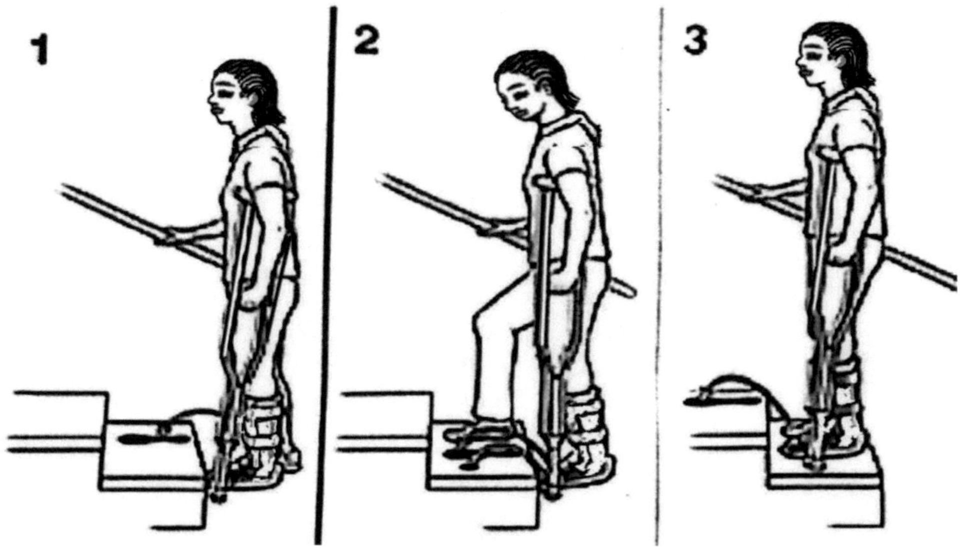

Figure 10.
Crutch placement (to support the affected limb) during stair case climbing using axillary crutches.

Axillary crutch	Height range
Pediatric	4′0″–4′6″
Youth	4′6″–5′2″
Adult	5′2″–5′10″
Tall adult	5′10″–6′6″

Table 1.
Available standard crutch length.

6.4 Foot-head linear techniques

- 77% of height of user is estimated to predict axillary crutch length.
- 75% of height of user is estimated to predict axillary crutch length.
- Height of user minus 16 inches (40.6 cm) is estimated to predict axillary crutch length.
- 77% of height of user plus footwear (2.54 cm) is estimated to predict axillary crutch length.
- 75% of height of user plus footwear (2.54 cm) is estimated to predict axillary crutch length.
- Height of user with FW minus 16 inches (40.6 cm) is estimated to predict axillary crutch length.

6.5 Arm-span techniques

- 77% of arm span of user is estimated to predict axillary crutch length.

- 75% of arm span of user is estimated to predict axillary crutch length.
- Arm span minus 16 inches (40.6 cm) of user is estimated to predict axillary crutch length.
- Olecranon to Middle Finger of other hand of user is estimated to predict axillary crutch length.

6.6 Foot-anterior axillary fold linear techniques

- Anterior axillary fold to heel of foot of user is estimated to predict axillary crutch length.
- AAF to heel of footwear (2.54 cm) of user is estimated to predict axillary crutch length.
- AAF to 15.2 cm lateral to heel of user is estimated to predict axillary crutch length.
- AAF to 15.2 cm lateral to footwear (2.54 cm) of user is estimated to predict axillary crutch length (**Table 2**).

	Correlation coefficient		
	r	r^2	*P*
Ideal ACL			
77% of height	0.951	0.904	0.00
75% of height	0.951	0.904	0.00
Height, 40.6 cm	0.951	0.904	0.00
77% of height + FW	0.951	0.904	0.00
75% of height + FW	0.951	0.904	0.00
Height + FW, 40.6 cm	0.951	0.904	0.00
77% of arm span	0.848	0.719	0.00
75% of arm span	0.848	0.719	0.00
Arm span, 40.6 cm	0.848	0.719	0.00
Olecranon to MF of other hand	0.835	0.697	0.00
AAF to heel of foot	0.967	0.935	0.00
AAF to heel of FW	0.967	0.935	0.00
AAF to 15.2 cm lateral to heel	0.967	0.935	0.00
AAF to 15.2 cm lateral to FW	0.968	0.937	0.00

ACL, axillary crutch length; FW, footwear; MF, middle finger; AAF, anterior axillary fold.

Table 2.
Prediction of axillary crutch length (courtesy [32]).

Elbow crutch	Height range
Youth	4′5″–5′5″
Adult	5′3″–6′2″

Table 3.
Available elbow crutch length.

The measurement of ideal axillary crutch length is measured in standing position. Potential user assumes a relax position (posture), measurement of a distance of 1.5–2 inches (3.8–5.1 cm) is made below the anterior axillary fold of the shoulder to a point 4–6 inches (10.2–15.2 cm) anterior and lateral to fifth toe of the ipsilateral limb.

Elbow crutch: this is also known as Lofstrand and Canadian crutch. It has the following components a single fore arm cuff (vinyl-coated, leather, plastic or rubber), a hand grip, and a single uprights vertical post (allow height adjustment) covered with a ferrule distally. The adjustment of the handgrip and upright bar are by using push button mechanism. The vertical bar is made of different materials such as wood, hard plastic, stainless steel, aluminum steel and iron.

Adjustment of height of the elbow crutch and the handgrip is standardized in an inch distance (2.54 cm). Adult elbow crutch range from 29 to 35 inches (74–89 cm). Only available in youth and adult range (**Table 3**).

6.7 Advantages

1. It is used to reduce weight bearing on one lower limb.

2. It is used to improve balance.

3. It is used to improve lateral stability.

4. It can be used for stair climbing.

6.8 Disadvantages

1. It need upper limb strength and coordination.

2. It need some trunk support.

3. It need good trunk stability.

6.9 Measurement for elbow crutches

The best position to estimate elbow crutches length is standing position. The measurement is from the tip of the elbow crutch at 4–6 inches (10.2–15.2 cm) anterior and lateral to fifth toe of the ipsilateral limb to the greater trochanter. The elbow crutches hand grip can be adjusted to allow elbow flexion of 20–30°. The forearm cuff is adjusted and positioned close to the elbow joint distally (proximal one third of the forearm).

6.10 Ambulation with crutches

The walking style a user of crutch will adopt is dependent on the medical condition, trunk control, balance, coordination, muscle strength, endurance, weight bearing status, functional capacity and learning ability. Prior to ambulation using crutches, the following safety and precautions should be checked:

- All the push button should be made visible and at same level.
- The ferrules should not be loose or worn out.
- The handgrips should be attached sturdily and not move when pressure applied.
- None of the component in the crutch should be loose.
- There should be no dents, cracks or any irregularities on the crutch.

The following instructions should be given to the users before usage:

- Users should maintain good posture (hyper flexion of the head, neck and trunk should be avoided).
- Users should avoid resting (i.e., bearing body weight) on the axillary pad.
- Users should avoid moving the crutches too far away during ambulation. The distance the crutch should be move should be within arm length.
- Axillary pads should be close to chest wall to improve lateral stability.
- Users should avoid pivoting when turning around, rather short circle movement should be used.

The following weight bearing status can be used with walkers: non-weight bearing (NWB), touch down weight bearing (TDWB), partial weight bearing (PWB), weight bearing as tolerated (WBT), full weight bearing (FWB) (**Table 4**).

Progression of axillary crutch walking is from non-weight bearing to partial weight bearing. Three-point gait first followed by four-point gait then two-point gait (**Figure 11**).

6.11 Standing from lying position with crutches

When in bed, the user first moves to a sitting position and maintain balance. The user then inches forward to the edge of the bed or the chair (users can also first transfer to an armless chair). The user picks up the crutches with upper limb of the affected side. Both axillary crutches are then placed upright and same side of the injured side. Using the armrest of the chair and the crutches handgrips as support, the user slowly moves the injured leg forward, moving out of the chair and rising up on the uninjured leg and the crutches. The user then position the crutches properly and then balances up in preparation to move, using any of the available weight bearing status that can be accommodated based on the user's condition.

6.12 Sitting with crutches

On getting to the chair, the user is instructed to turn and back up against the chair, moving backward until the back of the legs touches the chair. While bearing weight on the uninjured leg, and the crutches on either side of the user, the injured

	Non-weight bearing (NWB) and touch down weight bearing (TDWB)	**Partial weight bearing (PWB), weight bearing as tolerated (WBT) and full weight bearing (FWB)**	
	Three point axillary crutch gait	Four point axillary crutch gait	Two point axillary crutch gait
Pattern sequence	First move both axillary crutches forward and then weaker lower limb forward. Then bear all the weight down through the axillary crutches, and move the stronger or unaffected lower limb forward (**Figure 9**)	Left axillary crutch, then right foot, followed by right axillary crutch, and then left foot (**Figure 9**)	Left axillary crutch and right foot together, then the right axillary crutch and left foot together (**Figure 9**)
Advantage	Eliminates all weight bearing on the affected leg	Provides excellent stability as there are always three points in contact with the ground	Faster than the four point gait
Disadvantage	Good balance and coordination is required	Slow walking speed and difficult to learn	Can be difficult to learn the pattern
Progression	As the user becomes confident he may progress from a swing to gait to a swing through gait, where the unaffected leg is placed ahead of the crutches		

Table 4.
Ambulation with crutches [19].

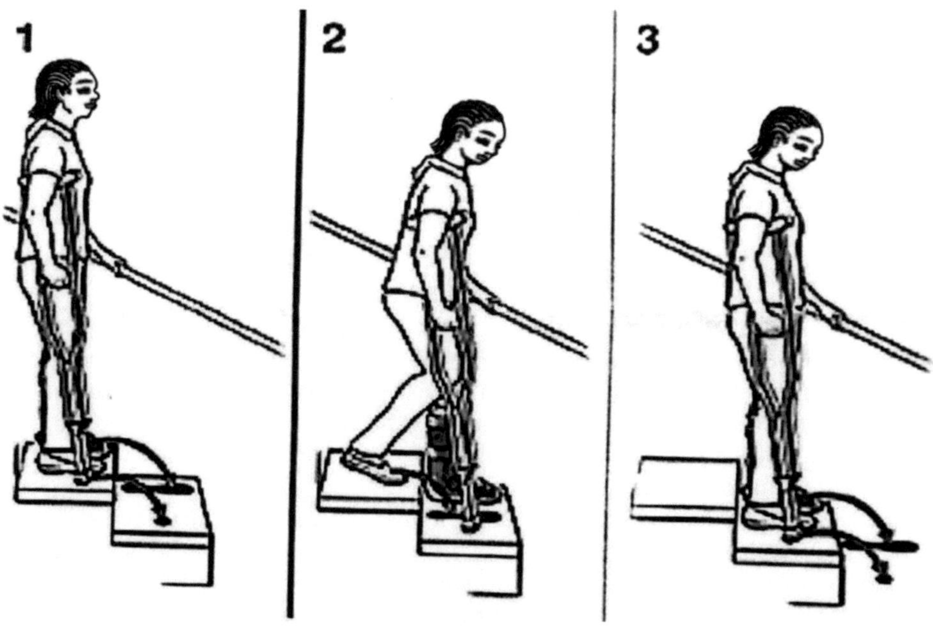

Figure 11.
Crutch placement (to support the affected limb) when descending stair case using axillary crutches.

leg is advanced slightly forward. Both crutches are rolled out of the axilla and held by the hand grip. Then, the crutches on the unaffected side is then moved across and on the outer border of the crutch on the affected side, such that both crutches are placed side by side on the injured side, and held at the hand grips. The user holds both handgrips together with the hand of the affected side and reaches back for the armrest of the chair with the other hand. Using the armrest of the chair and the crutch handgrips as support, the user slowly moves the injured leg forward and lowers himself into the chair. The axillary crutches are placed nearby. Standing them on the axillary pads, when possible, makes it less likely that they will tip over and fall away from the user.

6.13 Climbing upstairs with crutches

Climbing stairs with axillary crutches requires strength and flexibility. If the user is unsure of his strength, he should be instructed to turn around and sit on the stairs and scoot himself up one stair at a time using his uninjured leg to propel himself.

Where strength is available, the user is instructed to keep the axillary crutches in one hand and bring them up with him/her. When climbing stairs with axillary crutches, the user leads with the uninjured leg and brings the injured leg and axillary crutches up behind him (**Figure 10**). If the stairway has a handrail, the user should place both axillary crutches under the arm opposite the handrail and grip the handgrips together in one hand. The user places his weight on the handrail and the handgrips, leans slightly forward, and brings his uninjured leg up one step. He then brings the axillary crutches and the injured leg up the step and advances his hand up the handrail. Once the user has regained his balance, the process is repeated. The user should be instructed to take his time and rest halfway up the stairs if necessary. To climb stairs with no handrail, the user leans slightly forward and puts his weight on the handgrips of the axillary crutches. The user moves the uninjured leg up the step. He then shifts his weight to the uninjured leg and brings the axillary crutches and injured leg up the step. His foot and axillary crutch tips are kept in the middle of the step, away from the edge to avoid slipping. The user is instructed to take his time, rest as needed, and ask for help if necessary. Going up the stairs with axillary crutches stay with the affected leg behind and the uninjured leg goes up first.

Note that someone should always be at the back of the user learning to climb the stair with axillary crutches.

6.14 Going down stairs with crutches

Going down stairs with axillary crutches also requires strength and flexibility. If the user is unsure of his/her strength, he should sit down and scoot down the stairs one at a time, bracing himself with the unaffected leg. The user should keep the axillary crutches in one hand and take it along on the way down.

When going down stairs with axillary crutches, the user should lead with the affected/involved lower limb and the axillary crutches (the unaffected limb carries the whole body at this period) and then bring the unaffected lower limb down from behind (**Figure 11**) and then bring the unaffected lower limb down behind.

If the stairway has a handrail, the user should hold both axillary crutches at the hand grips and opposite the hand on the handrail. With the user's weight on the unaffected/uninvolved lower limb, the user moves the axillary crutches and the affected/involved lower limb down the stairs; with the user bearing weight on the handrail and the handgrips of the crutches and brings the unaffected/uninvolved lower limb down the stairs. The user should take time to regain balance. The process is repeated as the user moves forward. The users are given a prior instruction that they can rest when the need arises as they move down the stairs.

To go down the stairs with no handrail, the user bearing weight on the unaffected/uninvolved lower limb and the handgrips of the axillary crutches, moves the axillary crutches and the affected/involved lower limb forward down the stairs. The user keeps the foot and the tips of the axillary crutch at the middle of the step, away from the edge to avoid slipping. Are given a prior instruction that they can rest when the need arises as they move down the stairs. For safety reasons, someone (i.e., therapist) can walk in front of the users as they move down the stairs. This person can assist the user into a sitting position if users become fatigued. Going down the stairs with axillary crutches stay with the affected leg behind.

7. Cane

7.1 Description and components

Cane is also known as walking stick. It is a horizontal bar with a crook or T shape hand grip at one end and the tip (tips) covered by ferrule at the other end (**Figure 12**). The vertical bar is adjustable to fit the user. The vertical bar is made of different materials such as wood, acrylic, stainless steel, aluminum and iron. Most canes are usually between 25 and 40 inches long. Cane is typically used when minimal stability is needed and can support up to 25% of a user's weight [16].

7.2 Types

Standard cane: this is a single point straight cane with a crook or T-shaped handle.

Offset cane: this is similar to the standard cane but the proximal component of the horizontal shaft is offset anteriorly thereby creating a straight offset handle.

Quadripod: this is also similar to the standard cane, it however has a broad base of support with four point of support for floor contact. Others can come in form of a tripod.

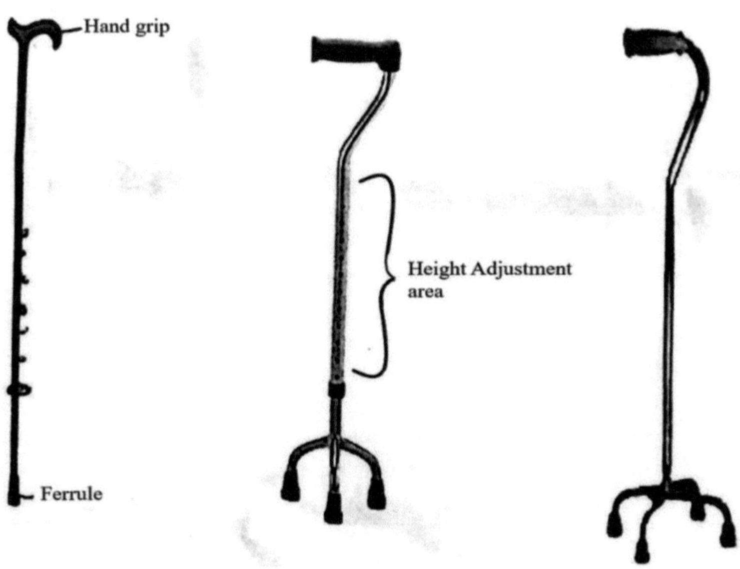

Figure 12.
Illustration of different types of cane—single point and multiple points.

Hemi cane: this also has four point of support for floor contact but the legs are angled from the shaft to increase stability of the cane.

7.3 Advantages

1. Cane is inexpensive.

2. Fit easily on every environment including stairs.

3. Use more for support than weight bearing.

7.4 Disadvantages

1. Not a good weight bearing ambulatory device.

2. Cannot be used by fearful user.

7.5 Fitting of cane for ambulation

The ideal cane measurement is obtained by placing the centre of the cane base at 6 inches lateral and anterior to the border of the fifth toe. Then the proximal part

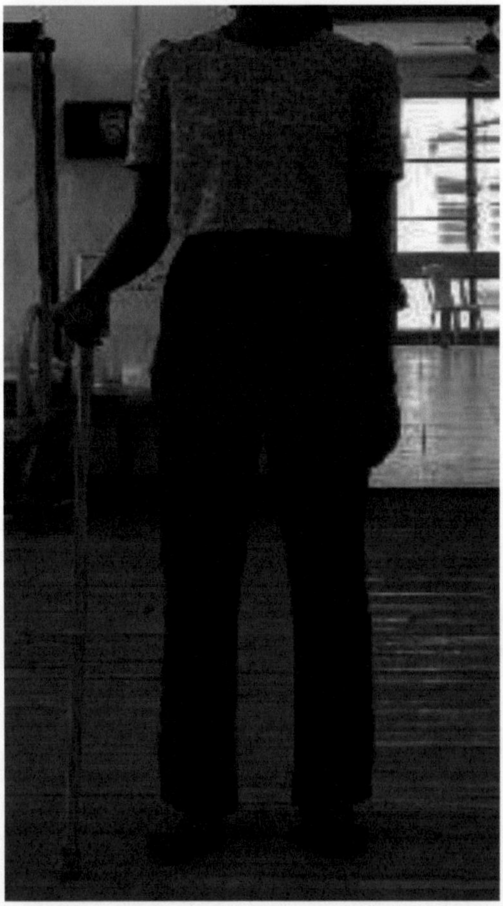

Figure 13.
Standing using the cane (full weight bearing).

(hand grip) at the level of the greater trochanter when the user is in an upright position. The user should have about 20–30° flexion of the elbow at this position (**Figure 13**).

7.6 Instruction on use of cans

It is usually advised to have the cane at the contralateral limb (i.e., opposite hemispace of the user for additional confidence). The user can perform 3-point or 2-point gait pattern with a cane:

3-point gait: the user first move the cane forward followed by the contralateral limb and finally the ipsilateral limb.

2-point gait: the user moves the cane and the contralateral limb together forward then the ipsilateral limb.

7.7 Maintenance of cane as an ambulatory device

1. The screw bolts and nut wings of the ambulatory device should be checked daily to be sure they are securely tightened.

2. Ferrules and wheels that become worn or tear should be replaced as the need arises.

3. Rubber handgrips that are torn or worn should be replaced promptly to prevent blisters on the hands or slipping of the hands.

4. Worn or torn rubber padding should be replaced to prevent pressure injuries.

7.8 Precautions when ambulating with ambulatory device

The following precautions are to be noted when ambulating with an ambulatory devices:

1. Items that may cause the user to trip and fall, such as scatter rugs or extension cords, should be removed.

2. Spilled liquids should be wiped up to avoid slipping.

3. Items the user needs with him can be carried in a fanny pack, apron with pockets, or knapsack to keep hands free to grip the ambulatory device.

4. A non-skid bath mat should be used in the shower or tub for users of ambulatory devices.

5. A tennis shoe or other flat, rubber-soled shoe should be worn on the user's uninjured foot to avoid slipping.

6. The user should be careful when going through doorways to be sure that the door does not shut on the ambulatory devices. The user should seek help to hold the door if necessary.

7. The user should avoid walking through water or on icy surfaces with an ambulatory devices.

7.9 Rules for safety and comfort when using ambulatory devices

The clinician needs to observe and check the followings:

1. Before issuing an ambulatory device the clinician should check that the ferrules (rubber tips) and wheels are not worn to the point where no tread is showing or not align. The ferrules and wheels are to act as friction and if they are worn out there is minimal friction and this is a potential risk factor for fall.

2. Ambulatory devices support areas are properly padded. This is important to avoid damage to soft tissues and provide comfort to the user.

3. Ambulatory devices pair is a matching pair. Clinician should not issue a mismatched pair. Uneven ambulatory device will lead to poor posture which can result into musculoskeletal disorder.

4. Ambulatory devices are not cracked, warped or damaged to prevent break of the ambulatory device and also prevent fall.

5. Ambulatory devices nuts and bolts are tight. This is important to avoid fall when the device is in use.

Users need to take note of the following rules:

1. User should not look down but always look straight ahead. This helps the user to maintain a good posture and prevent musculoskeletal disorders.

2. User should not use ambulatory devices when feeling dizzy or drowsy to prevent fall.

3. User should not walk on slippery surfaces to prevent fall.

4. User should avoid snowy, icy, or rainy conditions.

5. User should not put any weight on the affected foot if not advised.

6. User should make sure the ferrules (rubber tips) and wheels are present in ambulatory devices.

7. User should wear well-fitting, low-heel footwear.

8. Conclusion

Ambulatory devices are safe and promote users ability to function in activities of daily living when the right ambulatory device is prescribed and accurate measurements of users obtained prior to usage. It also reduces the burden of care and burden on caregivers. Trial and error method of prescribing and assessment should be avoided to prevent injury to the users.

Safety precautions should be observed by users and clinicians should always educate users on guidelines in ambulating with the devices and care of the devices.

Author details

Daniel Olufemi Odebiyi* and Caleb Adewumi Adeagbo
Department of Physiotherapy, College of Medicine of the University of Lagos, Lagos, Nigeria

*Address all correspondence to: femiodebiyi@yahoo.com

References

[1] Adegoke BOA, Maruf FA. Predictive ability of crutch-length-estimation techniques in apparently healthy university undergraduates. Nigerian Journal of Medical Rehabilitation. 2005; **10**(18):1-4

[2] Amaeze AA, Okoye GC. Analysis of method of axillary crutch measurement. Journal of Medical Research and Technology. 2006;**3**(1):27-31

[3] Arianne. Assistive Devices. 2004. Available from: www.everything2.com

[4] Bauer DM, Finch DC, McGough KP, Benson CJ, Finstuen K, Allison SC. A comparative analysis of several crutch-length-estimation techniques. Physical Therapy. 1991;**71**(4):294-300

[5] Beckwith JM. Analysis of methods of teaching axillary crutch measurement. Physical Therapy. 1965;**45**:1060-1065

[6] Bradley SM, Hernandez CR. Geriatric assistive devices. American Academy of Family Physicians. 2011; **84**(4):405-411

[7] Childress DS. Development of rehabilitation engineering over the years: As I see it. Journal of Rehabilitation Research and Development. 2002;**39**(6):1-10

[8] Clark BC, Manini TM, Ordway NR, Ploutz-Snyder LL. Leg muscle activity during walking with assistive devices at varying levels of weight bearing. Archives of Physical Medicine and Rehabilitation. 2004;**85**:1555-1560

[9] Crutch.com. History of Crutches. 2010. Available from: www.crutch.com

[10] Delisa JA, Cans BM, Walsh NE, Bockeneck WL, Frontera WF, Geiraingper SR, et al. Lower extremity orthosis, shoe and gait aids. In: Physical Medicine and Rehabilitation Principles and Practice. 4th ed. Philadelphia: Lippincott Williams and Walkins; 2005. p. 1391

[11] Dreeben-Irimia O. Assistive devices and gait training. In: Introduction to Physical Therapy for Physical Therapist Assistants. 1st ed. Sudbury: Jones and Bartlett Learning, LLC; 2007. pp. 246-247

[12] Emedicinehealth. Crutches. 2010. Available from: www.emedicinehealth.com

[13] Faruqui SR, Jaeblon T. Ambulatory assistive devices in orthopaedics: Uses and modifications. Journal of the American Academy of Orthopaedic Surgeon. 2010;**18**(1):41-50

[14] Feldman DR, Vujic I, McKay D, Callcott F, Uflacker R. Crutch-induced axillary artery injury. Cardiovascular and Interventional Radiology. 1995;**18**: 295-299

[15] Foot Health Facts. Instructions for Using Crutches. 2019. Available from: www.foothealthfacts.org/conditions/crutch-use

[16] Fulk GD, Schmitz TJ. Ambulatory assistive devices: Types, gait patterns and locomotor training. In: Physical Rehabilitation. 6th ed. Philadelphia: FA Davis Company; 2014. pp. 464-484

[17] Goh JCH, Toh SL, Bose K. Biomechanical study on axillary crutches during single-leg swing-through gait. Prosthetics and Orthotics International. 1986;**10**:89-95

[18] Hoeing H. Assistive Technology and Mobility Aids for the Older Patient with Disability. 2004. Available from: www.annalsoflongtermcare.com

[19] Inverarity L. How to Walk Safely with Crutches. 2005. Available from: www.physicaltherapy.about.com

[20] Kang YC, Choi EH, Hwang SM, Lee WS, Lee SH, Ahn SK. Acne mechanica due to an orthopaedic crutch. Cutis. 1999;**64**:97-98

[21] Kedlaya D, Kuang T. Assistive Devices to Improve Independence. 2008. Available from: www.emedicine.medscape.com

[22] LeBlanc MA, Carlson LE, Nauenberg T. A quantitative comparison of four experimental axillary crutches. American Academy of Orthotists and Prosthetists. 1993;**5**(1): 20-28

[23] Li S, Armstrong CW, Cipriani D. Three-point gait crutch walking: Variability in ground reaction force during weight bearing. Archives of Physical Medicine & Rehabilitation. 2001;**82**:86-92

[24] Lowman EW, Rusk HA. Self help devices, crutch prescription: Measurement. Postgraduate Medicine. 1962;**31**:303-305

[25] Martelli ME. Crutches and crutch walking. Encyclopedia of Nursing and Allied Health. 2010. Available from: www.findarticles.com

[26] McFall B, Arya N, Soong C, Lee B, Hannon R. Crutch induced axillary artery injury. The Ulster Medical Journal. 2004;**73**(**1**):50-52

[27] Mohammed-Arshadh YSK Munawar Physioheal. 2009. Available from: www.munawarphysioclinic.blogspot.com

[28] Monahan JJ. Mechanical therapeutic (casts, splints, tractions). In: Orthopaedics in Primary Care. 3rd ed. Philadelphia: Lippincott Williams and Wilkins; 1999. pp. 297-320

[29] Mullis R, Dent RM. Crutch length: Effect on energy cost and activity intensity in non-weight-bearing ambulation. Archives of Physical Medicine and Rehabilitation. 2000; **81**(5):569-572

[30] Najdeski P. Crutch measurement from the sitting position. Physical Therapy. 1977;**57**:826-827

[31] Nyland J, Bernasek T, Markee B, Dundore C. Comparison of the easy strutter functional orthosis system and axillary crutches during modified 3-point gait. Journal of Rehabilitation and Development. 2004;**41**(2):195-206

[32] Odebiyi DO, Adeagbo CA, Awe AG. Identification of axillary crutch length estimates that best predicts the ideal axillary crutch length in apparently healthy individuals. Journal of Prosthetics and Orthotics. 2016;**28**(**1**): 38-43

[33] Pariziale J, Daniels J. The mechanical performance of ambulation using spring loaded axillary crutches. American Journal of Physical Medicine and Rehabilitation. 1989;**68**(4):193-195

[34] Pierson FM. Principles and Techniques of Patient Care. Philadelphia: WB Saunders Company; 1994. pp. 106-109

[35] Poddar SB, Gitelis S, Heydemann PT, Piasecki P. Bilateral predominant radial nerve crutch palsy. Clinical Orthopaedics and Related Research. 1993;**297**:245-246

[36] Raikin S, Froimson M. Bilateral brachial plexus compressive neuropathy (crutch palsy). Journal of Orthopaedic Trauma. 1997;**11**(2):136-137

[37] Sadowski CA, Jones CA. Ambulatory assistive devices. Pharmacy Practice. 2014;**1**(10):24-31

[38] Salminen A, Brandt A, Samuelsson K, Toytari O, Malmivaara A. Mobility devices to promote activity and participation: A systematic review. Journal of

Rehabilitation Medicine. 2009;**41**: 697-706

[39] Schmitz TJ. Physical Rehabilitation Assessment and Treatment. 3rd ed. Philadelphia: FA Davis Company; 1994. p. 267

[40] Schoen DC. Musculoskeletal trauma, immobility and ambulation. In: Adult Orthopaedic Nursing. 3rd ed. Philadelphia: Lippincott Williams and Walkins; 2000. pp. 104-106

[41] Shortell D, Kucer J, Neeley WL, LeBlanc M. The design of a compliant composite crutch. Journal of Rehabilitation Research and Development. 2001;**38**(1):23-32

[42] Smith CP. Orthopaedics and trauma. In: Surgical Short Cases for the MRCS Clinical Examination. Revised ed. Cheshire: PasTest Ltd; 2002. pp. 245-246

[43] Subramony SH. Electrophysiological findings in crutch palsy. Electromyography and Clinical Neurophysiology. 1989;**29**(5): 281-285

[44] Thomas JM, Deshmukh N. Aneurysm of the brachial artery with complete thrombosis caused by a crutch. The American Surgeon. 1973;**39** (7):389-399

[45] Thomson A, Skinner A, Piercy J. Tidy's Physiotherapy. 12th ed. Oxford: Butterworth-Heinemann; 1991. pp. 437-440

[46] Van Hook FW, Demonbreun D, Weiss BD. Ambulatory devices for chronic gait disorders in the elderly. American Family Physician. 2003;**67**(8): 1717-1724

[47] Veerendrakumar M, Taly AB, Nagaraja D. Ulnar nerve palsy due to axillary crutch. Neurological Society of India. 2001;**49**(1):67-70

[48] Weiss RC. Assisting with ambulation and gait training. In: Physical Therapy Aide: A Work Text. 2nd ed. New York: Delmar Publisher; 1999. pp. 211-212

[49] Whittle MW. Pathology and other abnormal gait. In: Gait Analysis, an Introduction. 3rd ed. London: Butterworth-Heinemann; 2003. p. 111

[50] Wilson JF, Gilbert JA. Dynamic body forces on axillary crutch walkers during swing-through gait. American Journal of Physical Medicine. 1982; **61**(2):85-92

[51] Youdas JW, Brian MS, Kotajarvi J, Denny MS, Padgett J, Kaufman KR. Partial weight-bearing gait using conventional assistive devices. Archives of Physical Medicine and Rehabilitation. 2005;**86**:394-398

Chapter 6

The Argus II Retinal Prosthesis System

Edward Bloch and Lyndon da Cruz

Abstract

The field of retinal prosthetics has seen significant advances in the past 3 decades. Encouraging results from different groups have shown coarse objective functional improvement, using a range of technological and surgical approaches. The Argus II retinal prosthesis system was the first of its kind to receive regulatory approval for commercial use in Europe and the USA. The device is designed to replicate the function of photoreceptors in converting visual information into electrical neural signals in patients with profound visual loss secondary to degenerative retinal disease. Results from a phase II study of 30 patients have demonstrated improved performance in basic tests of visual function, object recognition, letter reading, prehension, orientation and mobility tasks. It is now the most widely implanted retinal prosthetic device worldwide. This chapter provides an overview of the requirements of a retinal prosthetic system, the results from the Argus II device to date, and an insight into some of the challenges and future directions of visually restorative therapies.

Keywords: retinal prosthesis, Argus II, artificial vision

1. Introduction

Retinal diseases, including both inherited and acquired conditions, are a major cause of blindness. In 2010, the WHO estimated that 285 million people in the world were visually impaired from all causes [1]. Hereditary retinal disease represents another significant contributor to unavoidable worldwide blindness, with conditions such as retinitis pigmentosa (RP) affecting an estimated 1/4000 people, or 0.025% of the population, often of working age [2]. Representing a heterogenous group of inherited diseases, RP affects the rod and cone photoreceptors (PRs), causing progressive, profound visual impairment, but with relative preservation of the inner retinal architecture [3]. This anatomical region consists of retinal ganglion cells (RGCs) and their nerve axons, which transmit visual information to the brain, along with other regulatory interneurons, such as bipolar, amacrine and horizontal cells, and Müller support cells (**Figure 1**). Preservation of these structures and the associated retinotopic map has led to RP becoming a model for many forms of visual restorative therapy, in particular, retinal prosthetics.

Another significant retinal cause of blindness is age-related macular degeneration (AMD), accounting for 5% globally [1]. It has been projected that, by 2040, this condition alone will affect 288 million people, 3.25% of the predicted global population [4, 5]. Late AMD comprises geographic atrophy (dry) and neovascular (wet) AMD, and is a significant cause of morbidity in the western world, with a

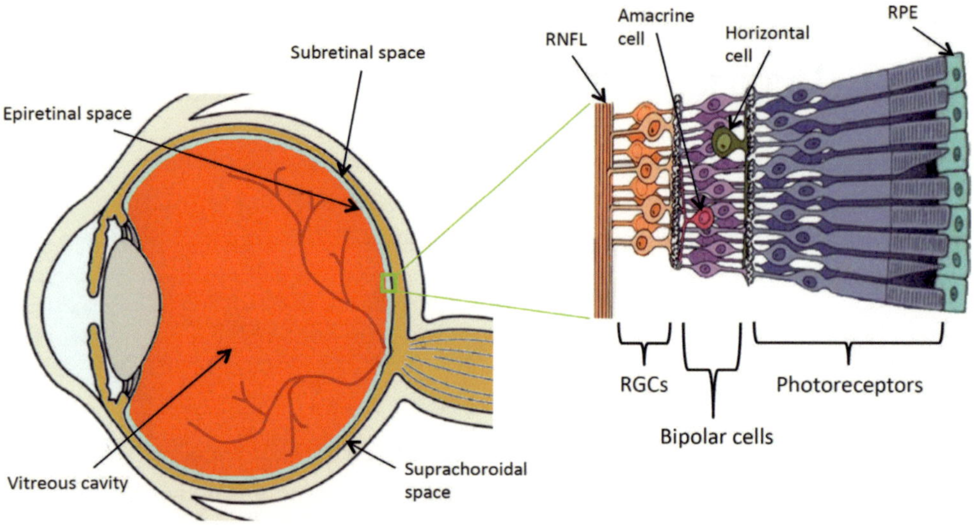

Figure 1.
A schematic demonstrating the anatomy of the eye and organization of the retina. RNFL: retinal nerve fibre layer; RGCs: retinal ganglion cells; RPE: retinal pigment epithelium.

prevalence of 2.4% in the UK [6, 7]. While anti-VEGF treatment has revolutionized the treatment of wet AMD, there is currently no treatment for the dry subtype, which results in degeneration of the PR layer and impairment of central vision in 1.3% of the UK population [7].

The concept of retinal prosthetics is centred on the phenomenon of electrically induced subjective visual percepts or 'phosphenes'. These phosphenes have been elicited by applying electrical currents across the ocular surface since as long ago as the eighteenth century. In the early twentieth century, Förster demonstrated that phosphenes could be elicited in blind patients via direct stimulation of the visual cortex, leading, in 1968, to the first chronic implantation of an intracranial visual prosthesis [8, 9]. In the 1980s, advances in microfabrication, materials engineering and retinal surgery provided a fecund environment for emergence of the field of retinal prosthetics—devices that could deliver direct stimulation to the residual retinal neurons.

2. Principles of natural vision

In order to create a *retinal* prosthesis, it is necessary to account for the processes that take place within the human eye, where light is absorbed, converted to an electrical impulse and encoded into a neural signal. Physiological capture of the visual scene occurs via the natural optical system, comprising the cornea, iris and crystalline lens, which focus light onto the photosensitive retinal cells. Within the photosensitive rods and cones, a photochemical reaction leads to transduction of light into a graded electrical neural signal with eventual RGC stimulation. The axons of the RGCs constitute the optic nerve. In the native retina, a significant amount of information compression occurs at the level the PRs, the interneurons and the RGCs, from where it is encoded for transmission via the optic nerve to the midbrain and cortical visual pathways.

There are two types of PR, rod and cone cells, which number ~120 and 6 million respectively in each eye, resulting in an average input of 100 photoreceptors to each of 1.5 million RGCs [10, 11]. Rods are sensitive to low levels of light and are most populous at about 20° eccentricity. The cone cells are responsible for colour vision and function best in bright light. They are most densely concentrated in the foveal region where they are in almost 1:1 ratio with RGCs, beyond which they decline considerably in density [12].

Following the transduction of photic energy into electrical impulses, bipolar cells effectively transmit the information from PRs to RGCs, but may have an excitatory (ON) or inhibitory (OFF) response to hyperpolarisation and are also influenced by the actions of horizontal and amacrine cells, which can introduce lateral inhibition of signals. Each RGC has a centre-surround receptive field organization and its stimulation pattern will depend both on the size of its receptive field, the input stimulation frequency, and whether it is an 'on-centre' or 'off-centre' cell. Furthermore, RGCs are not functionally homogeneous, with certain cell populations specialized in particular functions and projecting to specific midbrain regions. Most of the 1 million nerve axons of the RGCs pass via the optic nerve to their respective lateral geniculate nucleus (LGN), located within the thalamus. The LGN is a layered structure and each part receives axons from specific ganglion cell types. A degree of visual processing is thought to occur at this point, before projecting on towards the primary visual cortex, where all higher cognitive processing takes place [12].

The processing power of the retina enables us to resolve detail with remarkably high spatial and temporal resolution, across a broad spectrum of contrast and colour. Beyond this, higher neuro-cortical integration allows us to process and recognize objects, words and faces, appreciate distance, orientation and movement, while coordinating our visual interpretations with other sensory inputs and motor outputs. Together this information allows us to decide what is safe or dangerous, fast or slow, attractive or repulsive. All this activity occurs in milliseconds, with a seemingly infinite refresh rate. This phenomenon is reliant on a very complex system that can rapidly capture, assimilate, compress and process an enormous amount of visual information.

Clearly, creating a micro-electronic system, which can come close to replicating the processing capacity of the human visual system, is currently an unrealistic goal. Instead, we must focus on how visual processing software and hardware engineering can be combined to produce a device that can resolve the minimum interpretable visual information such as to be beneficial to patients with profound vision loss.

Simulated prosthetic vision (SPV) studies have been undertaken to try and estimate the optimum spatiotemporal image processing techniques for specific task completion, as well as the basic hardware requirements to best deliver RGC stimulation patterns [13–17]. SPV studies have extensively investigated the spatial resolution, visual field and contrast required for assorted activities of daily living, concluding that a minimum resolution of ~600–1000 pixels over a visual field 15° × 15° can permit reasonable accuracy in manipulation, recognition, orientation and mobility tasks. The resolution of around 3 pixels/degree^2 is similar to that in some currently available photovoltaic retinal prosthetic systems while fields of at least 15° × 15° have been created. However, and disappointingly, there remains a mismatch in the functional aptitude demonstrated by subjects in SPV studies and that in recipients of visual prostheses. This suggests that other factors, such as the effects of behavioural adaptation, perceptual learning and cortical plasticity, as well as the loss of the intrinsic retinal processing capacity, could be critical requisites in the development of a visual restorative system that could deliver appreciable functional value [18, 19].

One of the advantages of a *retinal* prosthesis is that, by placing a device at the most distal part of a non-functioning visual system, it is possible to benefit from any residual downstream neuronal organization within the retina and visual pathways. However this theory relies on the assumption that the proximal visual system remains intact. It has been demonstrated that outer retinal degenerative disease results in a cascade of reorganization and remodelling within the retina and central nervous system, even taking place before there is clinical evidence of PR loss [20–24]. A stepwise deterioration culminates in extensive neuronal cell migration, rewiring and death, accompanied by glial hypertrophy and retinal remodelling, rendering the retina incapable of processing or encoding visual data. This neuronal plasticity carries implications for all forms of visually restorative therapy, but particularly for prostheses, which are currently introduced at a late stage of visual impairment, where there has already been widespread reorganization with limited scope for rescuing vision. However, it may be that future iterations of bionic devices could even be introduced earlier in the disease process in an attempt to halt or reverse the remodelling process.

Another matter that remains unclear is the extent to which the human brain undergoes reorganization following loss of visual sensory input. Both animal and human studies have shown that there is the capacity for neuroplasticity as a functional adaptation to loss of a sensory modality [25–27]. For example, visual cortical activity has been demonstrated in blind subjects while reading Braille [28, 29]. Other studies of patients undergoing cochlear implant surgery, have shown correlation between the pre-operative auditory organization and activation and subsequent success of the neuroprosthesis [30, 31]. If a method could be developed by which a patient could be assessed for the feasibility of generating interpretable phosphenes, this would enhance patient selection and thus outcomes in this area of visual restoration. Further understanding of the nature of cortical plasticity in sensory loss and how subjects can adapt to a new form of vision with perceptual learning and rehabilitation, is sure to enhance the beneficial effect of visual restorative treatments in the future.

3. Principles of prosthetic vision

In order to simulate the complex series of events that take place between the outside world and the visual cortex, a prosthesis system needs to perform a specific sequence of actions, namely image capture, processing of the image, delivery of both image data and signal amplification to the microelectrode array, which in turn must deliver a suitable stimulation current (directly or indirectly) to the RGCs. All this must take place with a biocompatible system that can produce adequate stimulation currents without causing degradation to itself or to the target tissue. Furthermore, the device needs to be straightforward to implant, modify or explant, while remaining portable, discreet and fashionable.

3.1 Image capture

Presently, there are two principal means of 'image capture' that have found some success in retinal prosthetic systems. The first is to capture information from the visual scene using an external video camera, which is usually glasses-mounted. The video camera then transmits data directly to an external video-processing unit (VPU). The advantage of this approach is not only that it is technically simpler, but also it avoids any impediments to collecting high quality information about the visual scene, thus facilitating any downstream image processing. However, due to the fixed camera position, there is a risk of discrepancy between its orientation and that of the eye, risking inaccuracies in the perceived spatial location of an object of interest following retinal stimulation. Proposed solutions to this problem include both the incorporation of an eye tracker to coordinate the direction of gaze with the stimulation pattern, or placement of the camera system intraocularly, for which there have been some preliminary attempts to design such a system [32].

The second image capture system that has shown promise is the photodiode array device. First developed by the Chow brothers as the artificial silicon retina (ASR), this comprises a passive microphotodiode array, which was intended to intrinsically transform ambient light that falls on it into an electrical current capable of stimulating retinal neurons. The ASR array consists of 5000 interconnected photodiode anodes with individual isolated cathodes, each with an iridium oxide electrode. This method was advantageous in as far as it allowed a large number of pixels to be stimulated simultaneously, it was wireless and also it allowed for precise coordination between the eye position and the projected visual scene [33, 34]. However, in its first iteration, it was unable to deliver sufficient stimulation current to deliver functional results and the parent company, *Optobionics*, has since closed down. Despite this initial failure, the concept of the photovoltaic array has been taken up and developed by other groups, with encouraging results. The *Retina Implant AG* group developed the Alpha IMS device that contains 1500 independent and autonomous photodiode-amplifier-electrode units. The ambient light creates the stimulation pattern and an external power source amplifies the electrical signal [35, 36]. The 'PRIMA' Photovoltaic Retinal Implant system (*Pixium Vision* S.A.) combines aspects of both forms of image capture, in that is uses an external camera to capture the visual information before processing and then transmitting the data as pulsed near-infrared light patterns from a specialized visual interface in a pair of glasses directly onto a subretinal photovoltaic array [37, 38].

3.2 Image processing

In some systems, the image processing takes place within an external analyser, which receives a high-quality signal from a camera system and transforms the data into a set of commands to be wirelessly transmitted to the microelectrode array to generate a specific stimulation pattern. In systems such as the Argus II retinal prosthesis, there are only 60 microelectrodes, meaning that even with perfect electrode contact and accurate retinotopic phosphene perception, the image resolution would still be low. As such, there is an emphasis on developing software algorithms that can filter the most relevant parts of a visual scene, before creating simple stimulation configurations that map the object of interest onto the array. This process is known as saliency mapping, and similar algorithmic methods of rapid recognition and segmentation of information have previously been used with success in the form of speech processors for cochlear implants [39–42].

Simulation studies have shown that by applying transformations, such as edge detection, greyscale histogram equalization, intensity and contrast enhancement, task performance using a low resolution viewing system can be improved (**Figure 2**). Similarly, software has been developed to allow magnification of areas of interest in the visual scene, or even projection of a simulated object or face onto the array, in response to detection of the respective entity in the captured environment [43, 44]. The intelligent retinal implant system (IRIS) II (*Pixium Vision* S.A.) has a 'neuromorphic image sensor', which is designed to capture the coordinates and intensities of changing pixels, the information from which can be encoded and divided into transient and sustained components. This can be used to direct image processing towards the most relevant parts of the visual scene, i.e. moving people or vehicles, while removing redundant excess visual information [45].

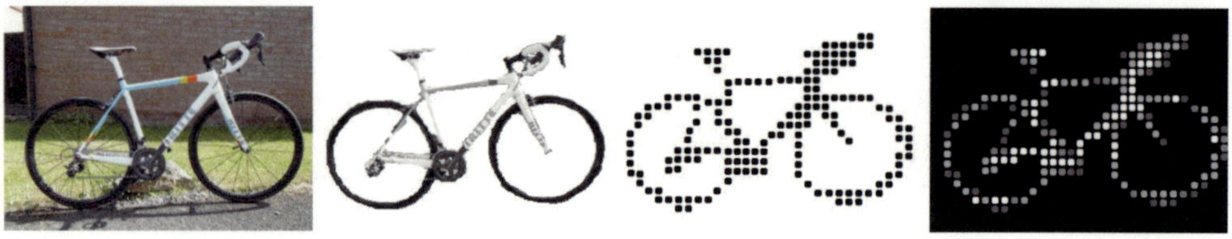

Figure 2.
An example of image processing transformations: the image of the bicycle first undergoes edge detection and is converted to greyscale. This is then transformed by circular binarisation into a black-and-white pixelated format. Finally the image is inverted, with the addition of four greyscale levels.

All these types of pre-processing are relevant for devices that do not have intrinsic photosensitivity, but instead rely on external image capture systems. In the case of the photovoltaic systems, there is a greater spatial resolution due to the high density of photodiode-amplifier-electrode units, each of which acts as an independent pixel. In theory, this enables greater intrinsic processing through more localized neuronal stimulation and may also incorporate some downstream processing from the residual retina to select and transmit the most salient visual information to the brain [46, 47].

3.3 Data and power transmission

Delivery of encoded visual information and power to the microelectrode array is generally either wireless (via inductively coupled coils) or directly onto the microphotodiode array via the natural optical system of the eye. In variations of the former approach, there are several considerations that need to be made. Inductive coil systems function through radio-frequency telemetry, whereby an AC current passing through the external coil induces an AC voltage in the internal coil, which can be subsequently be converted into DC power. A capacitor in series with the secondary coil permits amplification of the received voltage by creating a tuned resonance at the transmitter frequency, thus supporting efficient power transfer while minimizing the body's exposure to radiation. Although the data may be encoded onto the same signal as the power, it is more commonly accomplished with greater effect by using a separate, high frequency coil. The capacity for data and power transfer using this model is sufficient to support the resolution and refresh rate of current systems [48].

Location is an important consideration for an efficient inductive coil system. Many systems utilize a coil system that is similar to that of cochlear implants, with an electronics unit fixed to the bone postauricularly, which communicates with the retinal array via a tunnelled connecting wire. This approach was initially chosen due to the surgical familiarity to otolaryngologists and it allows for good coil contact for coupling. However, due to the prolonged duration of surgery, complex fabrication challenges and apparent reduction in system longevity, some systems have since been modified to incorporate a glasses-mounted transmitting coil which transmits to an implanted subconjunctival receiving coil, which is connected to the array via a sclerotomy. Another approach, as used in the EPI-RET3 implant, involves positioning a receiver coil into the lens capsular bag (following removal of the native lens). This approach still relies on an inductive power and data link, but negates the need for a transscleral wire, which carries a risk of infection and erosion. In addition, this system has a bi-directional enhancement system, which allows for simultaneous stimulation of and recording from the microelectrodes. Feedback from the system enables modification of the stimulation algorithms and patterns to accommodate any residual excitatory and inhibitory signal processing of the retinal neurons [49, 50].

3.4 Microelectrode array stimulation

There are several considerations when designing an electrode array to deliver electrical currents to the RGCs in order to replicate the spatial resolution (SR) of the natural retina. These include the electrode material, size, shape, spacing (pitch), tissue contact and the anatomical position of the array.

There are three primary sites for placement of a retinal stimulating microelectrode array (**Figure 1**): epiretinally (i.e. on the surface of the neurosensory retina), subretinally (i.e. between the retinal pigment epithelium and the degenerated outer retina) or suprachoroidally (i.e. between the sclera and the choroid). The advantage of the epiretinal placement is that the surgical approach is more familiar to vitreoretinal surgeons, allowing safer and easier implantation, adjustment and removal of devices. Furthermore, the interface with the vitreous cavity seems to permit safer heat dispersion. This set-up may be disadvantageous due to the fact that, in order to stimulate the RGCs, the stimulating current must pass through the retinal nerve fibre layer, which may produce ectopic visual percepts elsewhere in the retinotopic map.

In terms of a subretinal system, one proposed advantage is that by mimicking the position of the PRs in the natural retina, some of the stimulating current will pass via the residual bipolar system, exploiting graded response of the inner retinal neurons and thus the natural processing power of the retina. Moreover, it is felt that better electrode-tissue contact will be achieved with the subretinal than with the epiretinal approach. However, it has been noted that, due to underlying degenerative changes, surgical implantation can be difficult, and the longevity of these devices can be more limited [51].

Finally, suprachoroidal devices require a less invasive surgical procedure, which lends itself to easier repair or removal, but trials to date have been complicated by subchoroidal haemorrhage and fibrosis [52]. Due to the distance from the RGCs, these systems tend to require higher stimulation thresholds, leading to greater current dispersion and lowering the achievable SR. Overall, it seems that epiretinal and subretinal approaches have a superior performance in safety and efficacy to suprachoroidal implants. However, with pros and cons to both approaches, there is currently no clear evidence to suggest that, of these latter two, one system offers an overall advantage.

The challenge of electrode size and density is primarily a biological one, in as far as the native PR cells change in type, size, density and downstream signalling depending on their role and location in the retina. For example, cone PRs are, on average 6 μm in diameter, but in the centre of the fovea, they are around 1.5 μm in diameter and densely packed to permit the high resolution of vision that humans usually enjoy [53]. If we consider that normal vision is 20/20, meaning that the minimal angle of resolution at the retina is 1 arcminute, or the spatial frequency (SF) is 60 cycles per degree (cpd), then the SF required to achieve 20/200 (the approximate level of visual impairment) is 6 cpd. Since each degree angle subtended at the human retina is represented by ~280 μm, a SF of 6 cpd would necessitate a maximum pixel size of about 50 μm and, in turn an electrode size and pitch of 25 μm [54, 55]. Therefore, before factors such as electrode contact, dissipation of electrical current or heat are even considered, there is a significant theoretical constraint on the scale of manufacturing required to achieve a resolution corresponding to a visual acuity of 20/200.

Among the smallest electrodes that have undergone human implantation to date are those of the alpha IMS, which are ~50 μm in diameter, with a 70 μm spacing, giving a theoretical maximum VA of about 20/250 [36]. Results have been reported of a grating VA of 3.3 cpd and optotype recognition acuity of 20/546 using this device [56]. The Argus II device has 200 μm electrodes separated by 525 μm, which suggests a theoretical maximum VA of 20/1600. The best result, with grating acuity, has been reported as 20/1262 (just over 1 cpd) with this system [57].

Electrode shape is a factor that may significantly affect the integration of the device by creating an environment where retinal tissue can migrate around the array and create a close interface. Arrays have been designed with sunken chambers or 'wells', into which the inner nuclear layer cells have been shown to migrate. Another approach is the three-dimensional pillar array, with protruding electrodes, designed to produce an intimate apposition between the array and the neuronal cell bodies without requiring excessive remodelling of the retina [58].

Size, shape and contact of the electrode at the tissue interface are all important considerations to improve SR, but also have implications to the charge density per unit area. As the electrode size becomes smaller, there is an exponential increase in concentration of the current, which can result in target tissue damage [59]. Therefore there is an onus on finding materials that can permit the charge-injection requirements of neural stimulation, while minimizing conduction of heat or inducing tissue degradation. In addition to this, they must be biocompatible, waterproof and remain operational over an extended lifespan. While the precise electrochemical properties of the electrode-electrolyte interface, the capacitance and charge injection limits of different electrode materials is beyond the scope of this chapter, it is worth noting that new technologies, such as nano-coating, nanotubes and conductive polymers are providing promising developments in electrode fabrication, which may offer significant advantages over the more traditional metallic designs, such as iridium, platinum or titanium-based electrodes [60–62]. The emerging field of tissue electronics, which is focused on the use of organic conductive and semi-conductive polymer alternatives to inorganic electronic systems, is rapidly advancing. Recently, long-term *in vivo* studies of a fully organic multi-layer device in rats have shown success in recovery of subcortical and cortical light responses, as well as improvements in visual behaviour [63, 64]. While current electrode devices achieve RGC stimulation by direct current injection to trigger action potentials, it appears that organic coupling occurs in a more physiological manner by modulating local neuronal neurotransmitter release through discretely varying the membrane potentials [65]. It is probable that approaches using conductive polymers, or other chemical photoswitches (e.g. photochromic molecules or photoactive nanoparticles) permit a more natural interaction with the residual neuronal environment, which, in theory, could achieve cellular resolution.

4. Argus II retinal prosthesis system

The Argus II epiretinal device (*Second Sight Medical Products Inc.*) was the first retinal prosthetic system to obtain CE marking (2011) and FDA approval (2013) for commercial use, and is the most widely implanted retinal prosthetic worldwide. Comprising external and implantable components, it utilizes camera-based image capture and VPU processing, with wireless data and power induction, transmitting stimulation commands to an epiretinally located microelectrode array (**Figure 3**).

The Argus II system is implanted using standard pars plana vitrectomy and scleral buckling procedures, and usually the surgery includes removal of the native lens. Following removal of the vitreous and posterior hyaloid face, a conjunctival peritomy is performed and the recti muscles are isolated to allow fixation of an encircling band containing the internal coil and in-built application-specific integrated circuit. A 5 mm sclerotomy is created for insertion of the 60-microelectrode array and the connecting cable. This lies flush on the epiretinal surface and is secured in place using a spring-loaded titanium tack (**Figure 4**). A scleral allograft (or similar alternative) covers the hermetically-sealed coil and electronics case, which is then re-covered by Tenon's capsule and conjunctiva, such that the internal components are invisible to the casual observer. To use the device, the external components are worn, including a glasses-mounted camera and external coil, and a portable VPU and power unit [57].

4.1 Development history

Throughout the 1990s, Humayun demonstrated that low current stimulation of dissected animal retinal tissue could produce localized retinal responses [66]. This was followed by acute epiretinal stimulation experiments of blind human volunteers, with various forms of retinal degeneration. It was shown that stimulation could elicit subjective phosphenes, which in many cases could be accurately

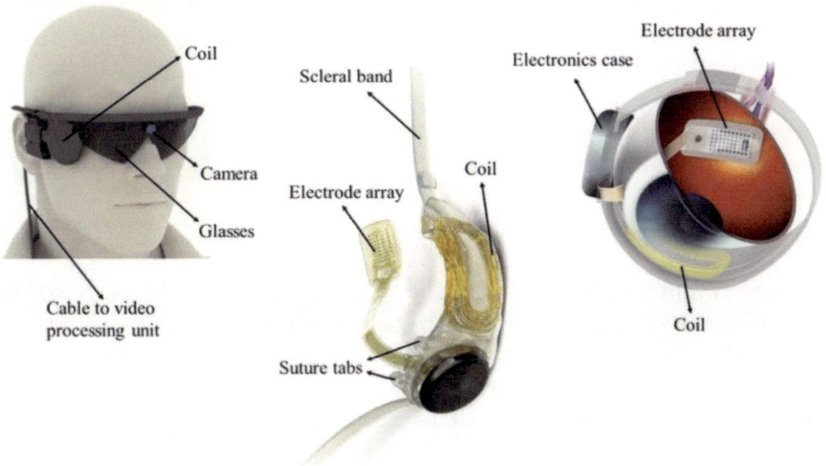

Figure 3.
The components of the Argus II retinal prosthesis system (adapted with permission from Second Sight Medical Products).

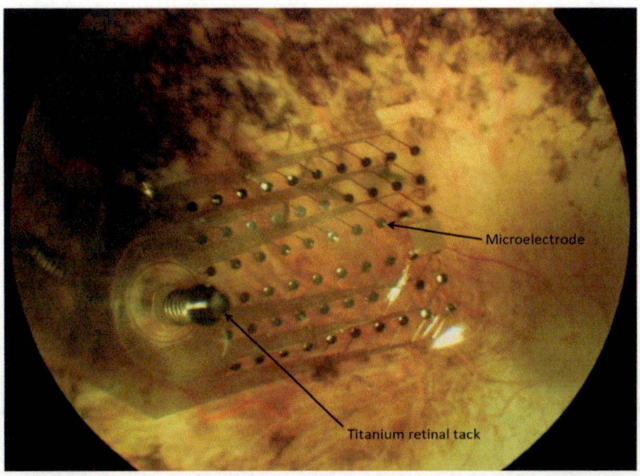

Figure 4.
Fundus photograph demonstrating an Argus II microelectrode array in situ.

localized and resolved to an equivalent acuity of up to 4/200 [67, 68]. In a subsequent series of acute stimulation tests using multielectrode arrays, two patients were able to identify crude forms from discrete patterns of electrical stimulation, using 400 μm electrodes arranged in 3 × 3 or 5 × 5 grids.

These promising results led to the development of the Argus I epiretinal prosthesis, which was the first device to undergo chronic testing in 2002 in six patients with end-stage RP. The Argus I device included a 4 × 4 array, comprising 16 alternating 250 and 500 μm diameter electrodes. The initial device design was based closely on that of cochlear implants, with an electronic unit surgically positioned in a postauricular recess of the temporal bone, from where a connecting cable would be passed along a groove in the bone and communicate with the intraocularly placed array. The external camera and VPU components captured the images, which, once encoded, were wirelessly transmitted via an antenna, that was magnetically held in position over the internal electronic unit. Results showed coarse functional performance was better than chance with the device on, with one patient able to detect light, motion and simple shapes [69–71]. In another subject, it was recently shown that the device continued to elicit phosphenes sufficient to permit target localization, orientation and mobility performance better than chance with the device on, 10 years postimplantation [72]. The overall safety and longevity of the device, which demonstrated coarse functional outcomes at a safe charge density limit, led to the development of the Argus II system, with a 6 × 10 microelectrode array and an optimized surgical approach.

4.2 Argus II results

The phase II multicenter clinical trial for the Argus II retinal prosthesis system began in 2006, enrolling 28 patients with end-stage RP, one with Leber congenital amaurosis and one with choroideremia. The primary endpoints of this study were safety and visual function, while secondary assessments of functionality included activities of daily living, such as orientation and mobility [57, 73, 74].

4.3 Safety outcomes

Witinn 12 months of the start of the trial, there were 18 reported serious adverse events (SAEs) requiring intervention, occurring in 10 of the 30 implanted patients. These included three cases of presumed endophthalmitis, three cases of conjunctival dehiscence, three cases of conjunctival erosion, two cases of hyptony, two arrays requiring re-tacking and one case each of rhegmatogenous retinal detachment, tractional retinal detachment, a retinal tear, corneal opacification and an inflammatory uveitis. The majority of these SAEs (78%) took place within the first 6 months after implantation and they were clustered among the initial 15 patients (72%). The reduction in SAEs in the second half of the trial was ascribed to refinement of both the device and the implantation procedure during the study, such as inclusion of prophylactic intravitreal antibiotics to the surgical protocol. All SAEs were successfully treated; in the cases of hypotony, the subjects required silicone oil tamponade (in one case for retinal detachment), which led to stabilization of the intraocular pressure [57, 73].

At 36 months, there were five additional reported late SAEs, including two further cases of hypotony and one each of infective keratitis, corneal melt and conjunctival erosion. Within this period, only one device required explantation, due to recurrent conjunctival erosion, and no eyes were enucleated [73]. At 5 years, the latest reported time point, there was only one additional SAE, which was a successfully treated retinal detachment, resulting in a total rate of 24 reported

SAEs among 12 (40%) of subjects. A total of three devices have been partially or completely removed at the request of the subjects, while a further seven subjects underwent elective repositioning during the trial to improve the contact of the array with the retina [74].

Overall, this is the largest and longest study of a retinal prosthesis system to date, demonstrating an acceptable safety profile and ongoing functionality and biocompatibility in the majority of subjects. Subsequent case series have shown improved safety profiles in parallel with growing surgical familiarity.

4.4 Functional outcomes

4.4.1 Visual function

There were three objective assessments used to evaluate visual function in the study. Firstly, a 'square localization' task, which involved the subject locating a white square displayed on a black background, indicated by touching the monitor. At 1 year, 94% of subjects could perform the task better with the device on than off. This was maintained at 3 years (89%) and 5 years (80.9%). The second task was 'direction of motion', which was assessed by asking the subject to indicate the direction of a high-contrast white line as it moved across the monitor. Initially 57% of subjects performed better than chance with the device on, which was once again maintained at 3 and 5 years (56 and 50%), respectively. Of note, these two tests of visual function were not performed in all subjects at the 1-year time point, due to their introduction partway through the study. Finally visual function was assessed using, 'grating visual acuity', which consisted of randomly generated widths of black and white gratings in one of four different orientations, displayed for 5 s on a screen. Throughout the study, 27–48% of patients scored better than 2.9 logMAR equivalent (mean 2.5 logMAR), depending on time point, with 38% performing significantly better with the device on than off at year 5. The best result recorded grating acuity was 1.8 logMAR, which approximates to a Snellen acuity of 20/1262 [57, 73–75]. The results from these tests of visual function are presented in **Figure 5**.

Dorn et al. tested the effect of providing scrambled spatial information to the device compared to one-to-one mapping, to investigate the degree to which the synchronization of multiple electrode stimulation conferred a benefit during motion detection. They found that of the 15 subjects who were able to perform the initial motion detection task better with the device on, 10 (67%) also performed better with one-to-one mapping of spatial information, than with scrambled information [76]. This suggests that the pattern of phosphenes being elicited was important for motion detection, and not that the patient was using the device to detect light, and simply scanning with their head to determine direction.

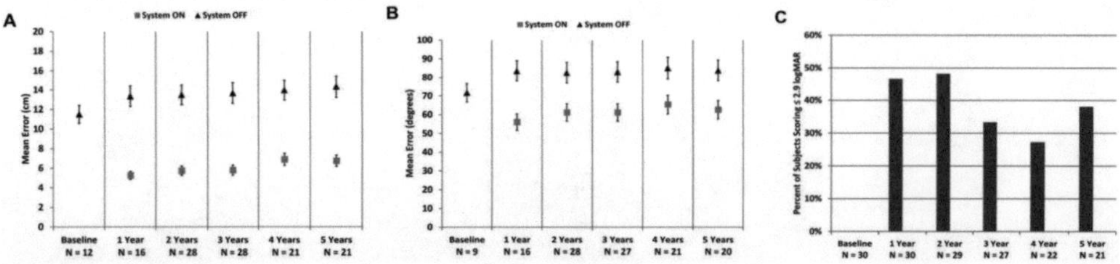

Figure 5.
Results for square localization (A), direction of motion (B) and grating visual acuity (C) at yearly time-points. Credit: da Cruz et al. [74].

4.4.2 Orientation and mobility

In the phase II clinical trial, two tests of orientation and mobility were employed. The first involved locating a simulated black door on a white background across the room. The second consisted of the subject following a 6-inch-wide white line on the floor, either configured as a straight line, or with a 90° turn along its length. Successful performance was maintained at ~50 and 70% in each respective task with the device on, which was significantly better than 15–30% success with the device off [57, 73, 74]. Dagnelie et al. found a similar rate of performance success using a real world 'sidewalk tracking' test in 27 implanted subjects, showing that 67% performed above chance with the device on, compared to 22% with the system off [77]. **Figure 6** illustrates the testing environments for orientation and mobility tasks.

4.4.3 Shape and object recognition

Arsiero et al. demonstrated, among implanted subjects, recognition of eight simple, solid, white shapes on a black background was significantly better the device on (31%) than off (13%), which improved further to 57% when the shapes were presented as outlines [79]. Luo et al. built upon this, presenting seven implanted subjects with eight high-contrast everyday items, both in the solid and outlined forms. It was found that subjects could identify solid objects to the same degree of accuracy with the device on as they could with the device on in the scrambled mode. Although superior to having the device off, this suggested that subjects were relying on visual cues other than the form presented but the array stimulation pattern. When the shapes were presented in their outlined forms, this significantly improved performance with the device on, above either that of the scrambled mode or with the device off [80].

Another real-world task described by Dagnelie et al., consisted of a 'sock sorting' task, in which subjects were asked to sort a randomly arranged collection of 10 black, 10 white and 10 grey socks into separate piles, according to colour. Each test was performed on a wooden table, or on a background of the subject's choice (i.e. black or white). In both scenarios, the subjects performed significantly better on average with the device on than off [77].

4.4.4 Letter reading

In a study of 21 implanted subjects, da Cruz et al. studied functional form vision by assessing ability to discriminate high-contrast letters. Letters were grouped according to typographical complexity and randomly displayed on a computer

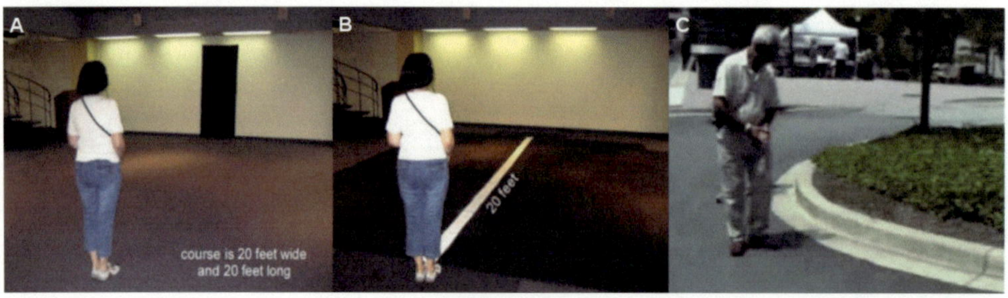
A
B
C
course is 20 feet wide
and 20 feet long
20 feet

Figure 6.
Photographs of subjects performing door finding (A), line tracking (B) and sidewalk tracking (C) tasks. Credit: Humayun et al. [78], Dagnelie et al. [77].

screen. Measurements from all subjects revealed a correct identification of 72% of group A (least complex) letters, presented at 30 cm, such that they subtended a visual angle of 41.27°. In the study, 19 and 20 subjects respectively completed the group B and group C letters, correctly identifying 55 and 52% in each instance. In all cases, performance was significantly better with the device turned on than off. A subset of six subjects who identified more than 50% of group A letters in fewer than 60 s went on to complete tests to assess the minimum letter size that could be resolved, while four of these six subjects were also assessed for performance on 2-, 3- and 4-letter word identification. The minimum letter size correctly identified was 0.9 cm, subtending a visual angle of 1.7°. On average, four subjects could identify 6.8 out of 10 words, ranging from 11 to 20 cm in height. In all cases, the performance was significantly better when the device was switched on in standard mode, than when scrambled or off [81]. These results are very promising for the capacity of some patients to achieve good spatial resolution, approaching the theoretical limit of the system.

4.4.5 Prehension tasks

In a series of experiments using a 3D motion-capture system, Luo et al. measured the ability of five subjects to grasp a white block on a black table (**Figure 7**). With the device turned on, subjects would successfully initiate and complete a grasping action 74% of the time, compared to 0% with the device off [82, 83]. Unlike other object recognition tasks, this study suggests a good capacity for the system to permit performance of hand-eye coordination tasks in a 3D environment, similar to that of the real-world.

4.5 Patient-reported outcomes

An important consideration in visual restoration is the extent to which the recipients judge the system to be beneficial in everyday life. The Functional Low-vision Observer Rated Assessment (FLORA) was developed by Geruschat et al. in order to evaluate the impact of partial restoration of ultra-low vision in subjects undergoing Argus II implantation. Initial results using the FLORA tool demonstrated that it was able to provide useful information about the everyday functional benefit of prosthesis-derived visual restoration, as well as identifying areas in which rehabilitation could be utilized to maximize subjective value. At 1 year, the assessment demonstrated an 80% reported positive effect, which dropped to 65% at 3 years. No patients reported a negative effect using this self-reporting tool [84, 85].

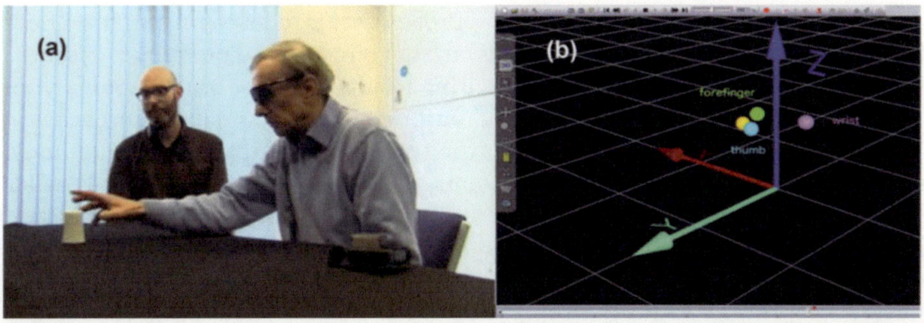

Figure 7.
Subject performing prehension task (a) with live infrared motion capture of subject's hand (b). Credit: Luo et al. [82].

5. Future directions

There are several other groups across the world using a variety of techniques to develop retinal prosthetic systems. Currently the intelligent retinal implant system (IRIS) II (*Pixium Vision S.A. France*) is the only other *epiretinal* device that has received CE approval. The external components and power induction mechanism of this system are fairly similar to the Argus II system. However, unlike the Argus II system, the 150-microelectrode array receives stimulation commands directly from an infrared array, which is integrated into a glasses-mounted visual interface, thus facilitating high data transfer and device miniaturization [45]. While initial data from the clinical trial were promising for functional and safety outcomes with the IRIS II, the study was postponed following concerns about device longevity [86].

The aforementioned Alpha IMS and its successor, the Alpha AMS (*Retina Implant AG, Germany*), have both been approved for commercial use in Europe. Utilizing photovoltaic technology, the Alpha IMS has 1500 autonomous photodiode complexes, giving a higher theoretical resolution than the Argus II. To date, this system has yielded safety and functional results similar to the Argus II, albeit with inferior longevity, possibly due to the surgical approach, involving subretinal device placement and a tunnelled link to a postauricular coil for electromagnetic power induction [35, 36, 87]. Preliminary data from trials of the Alpha AMS report considerable improvements in the lifespan of this system.

Finally, the Photovoltaic Retinal Implant (PRIMA) bionic vision system (also *Pixium Vision S.A.*) is currently undergoing a safety and performance evaluation feasibility study [88]. This subretinal system comprises a modular array set-up with 1 mm-wide hexagonal chips, each containing 142 30 μm-thick pixel cells, each ~70 μm^2, which receive visual data from a visual interface as pulsed near infrared light. Multiple photodiodes in series are stimulated, generating sufficient current to polarize the adjacent neuronal tissue with a local concentric return to limit signal diffusion. This system is unique in that it is scalable through insertion of additional chips and does not require any direct transscleral delivery of power or data [37, 89, 90].

Several other groups are also investigating alternative methods of neural stimulation, including optic nerve, cortical and thalamic prostheses [91]. As increasing numbers of patient volunteers undergo implantation with these systems, more data will become available, thus guiding the optimal design characteristics for future generations of devices.

Advancements in visually restorative medicine are not limited to prosthetics, with other regenerative technologies, including stem cells, gene therapy and optogenetics, demonstrating exciting developments in the endeavor to treat blindness [92–97]. In particular, optogenetics, an approach that is focused on targeting microbial opsin (light-dependent ion channels) to surviving retinal neurons to rescue or restore visual function, has shown exciting results in *in vivo* animal and *in vitro* human studies [98–100]. In addition to the aforementioned organic approaches, these techniques are attractive insofar as they offer a biocompatible, autonomous and scalable alternative to inorganic systems, which could be administered earlier in the disease course as a rescue therapy. It is widely anticipated that these strategies will soon build on the initial success of synthetic prosthetics, or potentially complement them in the form of biohybrid implants.

The success of the Argus II is representative of the enormous progress that has been made in the field of retinal prosthetics over the past 3 decades. However, there remain significant challenges to be overcome before the concept of 'bionic vision' is fully realized. Despite this, retinal prostheses have delivered the most compelling form of artificial vision to date, bearing testimony to the value of close collaboration between engineers, clinicians, patients and industry in pushing the boundaries of what is conceivable, let alone scientifically feasible.

Conflict of interest

The authors declare no potential conflicts of interest or financial support with respect to the authorship and/or publication of this chapter.

Author details

Edward Bloch[1,2*] and Lyndon da Cruz[1,2]

1 Wellcome EPSRC Centre for Interventional and Surgical Sciences, University College London, UK

2 NIHR Biomedical Research Centre, Moorfields Eye Hospital NHS Foundation Trust, London, UK

*Address all correspondence to: edward.bloch@gmail.com

References

[1] World Health Organization. WHO: Global data on visual impairments. 2010. Available form: www.who.int. (accessed 30 September 2018)

[2] Hartong DT, Berson EL, Dryja TP. Retinitis pigmentosa. The Lancet. 2006;**368**:1795-1809. DOI: 10.1016/S0140-6736(06)69740-7

[3] Santos A, Humayun MS, de Juan E, Greenburg RJ, Marsh MJ, Klock IB, et al. Preservation of the inner retina in retinitis pigmentosa. A morphometric analysis. Archives of Ophthalmology. 1997;**115**:511-515

[4] Wong WL, Su X, Li X, Cheung CMG, Klein R, Cheng C-Y, et al. Global prevalence of age-related macular degeneration and disease burden projection for 2020 and 2040: A systematic review and meta-analysis. The Lancet Global Health. 2014;**2**:e106-e116. DOI: 10.1016/S2214-109X(13)70145-1

[5] United Nations. UN: World population projected to reach 9.7 billion by 2050. http://www.un.org/ (accessed 30 September 2018)

[6] Jager RD, Mieler WF, Miller JW. Age-related macular degeneration. The New England Journal of Medicine. 2008;**358**:2606-2617. DOI: 10.1056/NEJMra0801537

[7] Owen CG, Jarrar Z, Wormald R, Cook DG, Fletcher AE, Rudnicka AR. The estimated prevalence and incidence of late stage age related macular degeneration in the UK. British Journal of Ophthalmology. 2012;**96**:752-756. DOI: 10.1136/bjophthalmol-2011-301109

[8] Foerster O. Beiträge zur Pathophysiologie der Sehbahn und der Sehsphäre. Journal für Psychologie und Neurologie. 1929;**39**:463-485

[9] Brindley GS, Lewin WS. The sensations produced by electrical stimulation of the visual cortex. Journal of Physiology (London). 1968;**196**:479-493. DOI: 10.1111/(ISSN)1469-7793

[10] Molday RS, Moritz OL. Photoreceptors at a glance. Journal of Cell Science. 2015;**128**:4039-4045. DOI: 10.1242/jcs.175687

[11] Curcio CA, Allen KA. Topography of ganglion cells in human retina. The Journal of Comparative Neurology. 1990;**300**:5-25. DOI: 10.1002/cne.903000103

[12] Purves D. Vision: The eye. In: Purves D, Augustine GJ, Fitzpatrick D et al, editors. Neuroscience. 5th ed. Sunderland: Sinauer Associates, Inc. 2012

[13] Dagnelie G, Barnett D, Humayun MS, Thompson RW Jr. Paragraph text reading using a pixelized prosthetic vision simulator: Parameter dependence and task learning in free-viewing conditions. Investigative Ophthalmology & Visual Science. 2006;**47**:1241. DOI: 10.1167/iovs.05-0157

[14] Sommerhalder J, Pérez FA. Prospects and limitations of spatial resolution. In: Artificial Vision. Vol. 519. Cham: Springer International Publishing; 2016. pp. 29-45. DOI: 10.1007/978-3-319-41876-6_4

[15] Sommerhalder J, Rappaz B, de Haller R, Fornos AP, Safran AB, Pelizzone M. Simulation of artificial vision: II. Eccentric reading of full-page text and the learning of this task. Vision Research. 2004;**44**:1693-1706. DOI: 10.1016/j.visres.2004.01.017

[16] Pérez Fornos A, Sommerhalder J, Pittard A, Safran AB, Pelizzone M. Simulation of artificial vision: IV. Visual information required to achieve simple pointing and manipulation tasks. Vision

Research. 2008;**48**:1705-1718. DOI: 10.1016/j.visres.2008.04.027

[17] Hayes JS, Yin VT, Piyathaisere D, Weiland JD, Humayun MS, Dagnelie G. Visually guided performance of simple tasks using simulated prosthetic vision. Artificial Organs. 2003;**27**:1016-1028

[18] Beyeler M, Rokem A, Boynton GM, Fine I. Learning to see again: Biological constraints on cortical plasticity and the implications for sight restoration technologies. Journal of Neural Engineering. 2017;**14**:051003. DOI: 10.1088/1741-2552/aa795e

[19] Chen SC, Suaning GJ, Morley JW, Lovell NH. Simulating prosthetic vision: II. Measuring functional capacity. Vision Research. 2009;**49**:2329-2343. DOI: 10.1016/j.visres.2009.07.003

[20] Jones BW, Watt CB, Frederick JM, Baehr W, Chen C-K, Levine EM, et al. Retinal remodeling triggered by photoreceptor degenerations. The Journal of Comparative Neurology. 2003;**464**:1-16. DOI: 10.1002/cne.10703

[21] Marc RE, Jones BW, Watt CB, Strettoi E. Neural remodeling in retinal degeneration. Progress in Retinal and Eye Research. 2003;**22**:607-655. DOI: 10.1016/S1350-9462(03)00039-9

[22] Cuenca N, Pinilla I, Sauvé Y, Lund R. Early changes in synaptic connectivity following progressive photoreceptor degeneration in RCS rats. The European Journal of Neuroscience. 2005;**22**:1057-1072. DOI: 10.1111/j.1460-9568.2005.04300.x

[23] Jones BW, Marc RE. Retinal remodeling during retinal degeneration. Experimental Eye Research. 2005;**81**:123-137. DOI: 10.1016/j.exer.2005.03.006

[24] Marc RE, Jones BW, Anderson JR, Kinard K, Marshak DW, Wilson JH, et al. Neural reprogramming in retinal degeneration. Investigative Ophthalmology & Visual Science. 2007;**48**:3364-3371. DOI: 10.1167/iovs.07-0032

[25] Ptito M. Cross-modal plasticity: Lessons from the visual system. Journal of Vision. 2006;**6**:11-11. DOI: 10.1167/6.13.11

[26] Merabet LB, Rizzo JF, Amedi A, Somers DC, Pascual-Leone A. What blindness can tell us about seeing again: Merging neuroplasticity and neuroprostheses. Nature Reviews Neuroscience. 2005;**6**:71-77. DOI: 10.1038/nrn1586

[27] Bavelier D, Neville HJ. Cross-modal plasticity: Where and how? Nature Reviews Neuroscience. 2002;**3**:443-452. DOI: 10.1038/nrn848

[28] Sadato N, Pascual-Leone A, Grafman J, Ibañez V, Deiber M-P, Dold G, et al. Activation of the primary visual cortex by Braille reading in blind subjects. Nature. 1996;**380**:526-528. DOI: 10.1038/380526a0

[29] Sadato N, Yonekura Y, Ishii Y, Deiber MP, Ibanez V, Hallett M. Neural networks for braille reading by the blind include visual cortex. NeuroImage. 1996;**3**:S340. DOI: 10.1016/S1053-8119(96)80342-9

[30] Giraud A-L, Lee H-J. Predicting cochlear implant outcome from brain organisation in the deaf. Restorative Neurology and Neuroscience. 2007;**25**:381-390

[31] Roland PS, Tobey EA, Devous MD Sr. Preoperative functional assessment of auditory cortex in adult Cochlear implant users. The Laryngoscope. 2001;**111**:77-83. DOI: 10.1097/00005537-200101000-00013

[32] Nasiatka P, Ahuja AK, Stiles N, Hauer M, Agrawal RN, Freda R, et al. Intraocular camera for retinal prostheses. Investigative

Ophthalmology & Visual Science. 2005;**46**:5277

[33] Chow AY. The artificial silicon retina microchip for the treatment of vision loss from retinitis pigmentosa. Archives of Ophthalmology. 2004;**122**:460. DOI: 10.1001/archopht.122.4.460

[34] Chow AY, Bittner AK, Pardue MT. The artificial silicon retina in retinitis pigmentosa patients (an American Ophthalmological Association thesis). Transactions of the American Ophthalmological Society. 2010;**108**:120-154

[35] Stingl K, Bach M, Bartz-Schmidt KU, Braun A, Bruckmann A, Gekeler F, et al. Safety and efficacy of subretinal visual implants in humans: Methodological aspects. Clinical & Experimental Optometry. 2013;**96**:4-13. DOI: 10.1111/j.1444-0938.2012.00816.x

[36] Stingl K, Bartz-Schmidt KU, Besch D, Braun A, Bruckmann A, Gekeler F, et al. Artificial vision with wirelessly powered subretinal electronic implant alpha-IMS. Proceedings of the Biological Sciences. 2013;**280**:20130077-20130077. DOI: 10.1098/rspb.2013.0077

[37] Lorach H, Palanker D. High resolution photovoltaic subretinal prosthesis for restoration of sight. In: Artificial Vision. Vol. 19. Cham: Springer International Publishing; 2016. pp. 115-124. DOI: 10.1007/978-3-319-41876-6_9

[38] Mandel Y, Goetz G, Lavinsky D, Huie P, Mathieson K, Wang L, et al. *In vivo* performance of photovoltaic subretinal prosthesis. In: Manns F, Söderberg PG, Ho A, editors. SPIE BiOS. Vol. 8567. San Francisco: SPIE; 2013. p. 856709. DOI: 10.1117/12.2001750

[39] Itti L, Koch C, Niebur E. A model of saliency-based visual attention for rapid scene analysis. IEEE Transactions on Pattern Analysis and Machine Intelligence. 1998;**20**:1254-1259. DOI: 10.1109/34.730558

[40] Wilson BS, Finley CC, Lawson DT, Wolford RD, Eddington DK, Rabinowitz WM. Better speech recognition with cochlear implants. Nature. 1991;**352**:236-238. DOI: 10.1038/352236a0

[41] Feng C, Dai S, Zhao Y, Liu S. Edge-preserving image decomposition based on saliency map. In: 2014 7th International Congress on Image and Signal Processing (CISP). IEEE; 2014. pp. 159-163. DOI: 10.1109/CISP.2014.7003769

[42] Parikh N, Itti L, Weiland J. Saliency-based image processing for retinal prostheses. Journal of Neural Engineering. 2010;**7**:016006. DOI: 10.1088/1741-2560/7/1/016006

[43] Stanga P, Sahel J, Mohand-Said S, da Cruz L, Caspi A, Merlini F, et al. Face detection using the Argus® II Retinal Prosthesis System. Investigative Ophthalmology & Visual Science. 2013;**54**:1766

[44] Thompson RW, Barnett GD, Humayun MS, Dagnelie G. Facial recognition using simulated prosthetic pixelized vision. Investigative Ophthalmology & Visual Science. 2003;**44**:5035-5042

[45] Hornig R, Dapper M, Le Joliff E, Hill R, Ishaque K, Posch C, et al. Pixium vision: First clinical results and innovative developments. In: Artificial Vision. Vol. 9. Cham: Springer International Publishing; 2016. pp. 99-113. DOI: 10.1007/978-3-319-41876-6_8

[46] Zrenner E, Bartz-Schmidt KU, Benav H, Besch D, Bruckmann A, Gabel VP, et al. Subretinal electronic chips allow blind patients to read letters and combine them to words. Proceedings of

the Biological Sciences. 2011;**278**: 1489-1497. DOI: 10.1098/rspb.2010.1747

[47] Wang L, Mathieson K, Kamins TI, Loudin JD, Galambos L, Goetz G, et al. Photovoltaic retinal prosthesis: Implant fabrication and performance. Journal of Neural Engineering. 2012;**9**:046014. DOI: 10.1088/1741-2560/9/4/046014

[48] Loudin JD, Butterwick A, Huie P, Palanker D. Delivery of information and power to the implant, integration of the electrode array with the retina, and safety of chronic stimulation. In: Dagnelie G, editor. Visual Prosthetics: Physiology, Bioengineering, Rehabilitation. New York: Springer Science+Business Media. 2011

[49] Schloesser M, Cota O, Heil R, Brusius J, Offenhausser A, Waasen SV, et al. Embedded device for simultaneous recording and stimulation for retina implant research. In: 2013 IEEE Sensors. IEEE; 2013. pp. 1-4. DOI: 10.1109/ICSENS.2013.6688173

[50] Walter P. A fully intraocular approach for a bi-directional retinal prosthesis. In: Artificial Vision. Vol. 2009. Cham: Springer International Publishing; 2016. pp. 151-161. DOI: 10.1007/978-3-319-41876-6_12

[51] Gekeler F, Sachs H, Kitiratschky VBD, Stingl K, Greppmaier U, Zrenner E, et al. Re-alignment and explantation of subretinal prostheses: Surgical aspects and proteomic analyses. Investigative Ophthalmology & Visual Science. 2013;**54**:1036

[52] Ayton LN, Blamey PJ, Guymer RH, Luu CD, Nayagam DAX, Sinclair NC, et al. First-in-human trial of a novel suprachoroidal retinal prosthesis. PLoS One. 2014;**9**:e115239. DOI: 10.1371/journal.pone.0115239

[53] Kolb H. Photoreceptors. In: Kolb H, Fernandez E, Nelson R, editors. The Organization of the Retina and Visual System. Utah: Webvision. 1995

[54] Cohen E. Retinal prostheses. In Kolb H, Fernandez E, Nelson R, editors. The Organization of the Retina and Visual System. Utah: Webvision. 1995

[55] Zrenner E. Fighting blindness with microelectronics. Science Translational Medicine. 2013;**5**(210):1-7. DOI: 10.1126/scitranslmed.3007399

[56] Stingl K, Schippert R, Bartz-Schmidt KU, Besch D, Cottriall CL, Edwards TL, et al. Interim results of a multicenter trial with the new electronic subretinal implant alpha AMS in 15 patients blind from inherited retinal degenerations. Frontiers in Neuroscience. 2017;**11**:445. DOI: 10.3389/fnins.2017.00445

[57] Humayun MS, Dorn JD, da Cruz L, Dagnelie G, Sahel J-A, Stanga PE, et al. Interim results from the international trial of second sight's visual prosthesis. Ophthalmology. 2012;**119**:779-788. DOI: 10.1016/j.ophtha.2011.09.028

[58] Butterwick A, Huie P, Jones BW, Marc RE, Marmor M, Palanker D. Effect of shape and coating of a subretinal prosthesis on its integration with the retina. Experimental Eye Research. 2009;**88**:22-29. DOI: 10.1016/j.exer.2008.09.018

[59] Butterwick A, Vankov A, Huie P, Freyvert Y, Palanker D. Tissue damage by pulsed electrical stimulation. IEEE Transactions on Biomedical Engineering. 2007;**54**:2261-2267

[60] Wang K, Fishman HA, Dai H, Harris JS. Neural stimulation with a carbon nanotube microelectrode array. Nano Letters. 2006;**6**:2043-2048. DOI: 10.1021/nl061241t

[61] Harris AR, Wallace GG. Organic electrodes and communications with excitable cells. Advanced Functional Materials. 2017;**28**:1700587. DOI: 10.1002/adfm.201700587

[62] Richardson-Burns SM, Hendricks JL, Foster B, Povlich LK, Kim D-H, Martin DC. Polymerization of the conducting polymer poly(3,4-ethylenedioxythiophene) (PEDOT) around living neural cells. Biomaterials. 2007;**28**:1539-1552. DOI: 10.1016/j.biomaterials.2006.11.026

[63] Ghezzi D, Antognazza MR, Mete M, Pertile G, Lanzani G, Benfenati F. A polymer optoelectronic interface restores light sensitivity in blind rat retinas. Nature Photonics. 2013;**7**(5):400-406

[64] Maya-Vetencourt JF, Ghezzi D, Antognazza MR, Colombo E, Mete M, Feyen P, et al. A fully organic retinal prosthesis restores vision in a rat model of degenerative blindness. Nature Materials. 2017;**16**:681-689. DOI: 10.1038/nmat4874

[65] Benfenati F, Lanzani G. New technologies for developing second generation retinal prostheses. Lab Animal. 2018;**47**:71-75. DOI: 10.1038/s41684-018-0003-1

[66] Humayun M. Bipolar surface electrical stimulation of the vertebrate retina. Archives of Ophthalmology. 1994;**112**:110-116. DOI: 10.1001/archopht.1994.01090130120028

[67] Humayun MS. Visual perception elicited by electrical stimulation of retina in blind humans. Archives of Ophthalmology. 1996;**114**:40-46. DOI: 10.1001/archopht.1996.01100130038006

[68] Humayun MS, de Juan E, Weiland JD, Dagnelie G, Katona S, Greenberg R, et al. Pattern electrical stimulation of the human retina. Vision Research. 1999;**39**:2569-2576

[69] Humayun MS, Weiland JD, Fujii GY, Greenberg R, Williamson R, Little J, et al. Visual perception in a blind subject with a chronic microelectronic retinal prosthesis. Vision Research. 2003;**43**:2573-2581. DOI: 10.1016/S0042-6989(03)00457-7

[70] Humayun MS, Freda R, Fine I, Roy A, Fujii G, Greenberg RJ, et al. Implanted intraocular retinal prosthesis in six blind subjects. Investigative Ophthalmology & Visual Science. 2005;**46**:1144

[71] Caspi A, Dorn JD, McClure KH, Humayun MS, Greenberg RJ, McMahon MJ. Feasibility study of a retinal prosthesis: Spatial vision with a 16-electrode implant. Archives of Ophthalmology. 2009;**127**:398-401. DOI: 10.1001/archophthalmol.2009.20

[72] Yue L, Falabella P, Christopher P, Wuyyuru V, Dorn J, Schor P, et al. Ten-year follow-up of a blind patient chronically implanted with epiretinal prosthesis Argus I. Ophthalmology. 2015;**122**:2545-2552.e1. DOI: 10.1016/j.ophtha.2015.08.008

[73] Ho AC, Humayun MS, Dorn JD, da Cruz L, Dagnelie G, Handa J, et al. Long-term results from an epiretinal prosthesis to restore sight to the blind. Ophthalmology. 2015;**122**:1547-1554. DOI: 10.1016/j.ophtha.2015.04.032

[74] da Cruz L, Dorn JD, Humayun MS, Dagnelie G, Handa J, Barale P-O, et al. Five-year safety and performance results from the Argus II retinal prosthesis system clinical trial. Ophthalmology. 2016;**123**:2248-2254. DOI: 10.1016/j.ophtha.2016.06.049

[75] Ahuja AK, Dorn JD, Caspi A, McMahon MJ, Dagnelie G, Dacruz L, et al. Blind subjects implanted with the Argus II retinal prosthesis are able to improve performance in a spatial-motor task. The British Journal of Ophthalmology. 2011;**95**:539-543. DOI: 10.1136/bjo.2010.179622

[76] Dorn JD, Ahuja AK, Caspi A, da Cruz L, Dagnelie G, Sahel J-A, et al.

The detection of motion by blind subjects with the epiretinal 60-electrode (Argus II) retinal prosthesis. JAMA ophthalmology. 2013;**131**:183-189. DOI: 10.1001/2013.jamaophthalmol.221

[77] Dagnelie G, Christopher P, Arditi A, da Cruz L, Duncan JL, Ho AC, et al. Performance of real-world functional vision tasks by blind subjects improves after implantation with the Argus® II retinal prosthesis system. Clinical & Experimental Ophthalmology. 2017;**45**:152-159. DOI: 10.1111/ceo.12812

[78] Humayun MS, Dorn JD, Ahuja AK, Caspi A, Filley E, Dagnelie G, et al. Preliminary 6 month results from the Argus II epiretinal prosthesis feasibility study. Conference Proceedings: Annual International Conference of the IEEE Engineering in Medicine and Biology Society. 2009;**2009**:4566-4568. DOI: 10.1109/IEMBS.2009.5332695

[79] Arsiero M, da Cruz L, Merlini F, Sahel J, Stanga P, Hafezi F, et al. Subjects blinded by outer retinal dystrophies are able to recognize shapes using the Argus II retinal prosthesis system. Investigative Ophthalmology & Visual Science. 2011;**52**:4951

[80] Luo YH-L, Zhong J, Merlini F, Anaflous F, Arsiero M, Stanga P, et al. The use of Argus® II retinal prosthesis to identify common objects in blind subjects with outer retinal dystrophies. Investigative Ophthalmology & Visual Science. 2014;**55**:1834

[81] da Cruz L, Coley BF, Dorn J, Merlini F, Filley E, Christopher P, et al. The Argus II epiretinal prosthesis system allows letter and word reading and long-term function in patients with profound vision loss. The British Journal of Ophthalmology. 2013;**97**:632-636. DOI: 10.1136/bjophthalmol-2012-301525

[82] Luo YH-L, Zhong JJ, da Cruz L. The use of Argus® II retinal prosthesis by blind subjects to achieve localisation and prehension of objects in 3-dimensional space. Graefe's Archive for Clinical and Experimental Ophthalmology. 2015;**253**:1907-1914. DOI: 10.1007/s00417-014-2912-z

[83] Kotecha A, Zhong J, Stewart D, da Cruz L. The Argus II prosthesis facilitates reaching and grasping tasks: A case series. BMC Ophthalmology. 2014;**14**:71. DOI: 10.1186/1471-2415-14-71

[84] Geruschat DR, Flax M, Tanna N, Bianchi M, Fisher A, Goldschmidt M, et al. FLORA™: Phase I development of a functional vision assessment for prosthetic vision users. Clinical & Experimental Optometry. 2015;**98**: 342-347. DOI: 10.1111/cxo.12242

[85] Geruschat DR, Richards TP, Arditi A, da Cruz L, Dagnelie G, Dorn JD, et al. An analysis of observer-rated functional vision in patients implanted with the Argus II retinal prosthesis system at three years. Clinical & Experimental Optometry. 2016;**99**:227-232. DOI: 10.1111/cxo.12359

[86] Muqit M, LeMer Y, De Rothschild A, Velikay-Parel M, Weber M, Dupeyron G, et al. Results at 6 months. Available from: www.pixium-vision.com [Accessed: 30 September 2018]

[87] Kitiratschky VBD, Stingl K, Wilhelm B, Peters T, Besch D, Sachs H, et al. Safety evaluation of "retina implant alpha IMS"—A prospective clinical trial. Graefe's Archive for Clinical and Experimental Ophthalmology. 2014;**253**:381-387. DOI: 10.1007/s00417-014-2797-x

[88] Pixium Vision: Dry AMD PRIMA. https://www.pixium-vision.com/ (accessed 30 September 2018)

[89] Lorach H, Goetz G, Smith R, Lei X, Mandel Y, Kamins T, et al. Photovoltaic restoration of sight with high visual

acuity. Nature Medicine. 2015;**21**: 476-482. DOI: 10.1038/nm.3851

[90] Mandel Y, Goetz G, Lavinsky D, Huie P, Mathieson K, Wang L, et al. Cortical responses elicited by photovoltaic subretinal prostheses exhibit similarities to visually evoked potentials. Nature Communications. 2013;**4**:564. DOI: 10.1038/ncomms2980

[91] Zrenner E, Greger B. Chapter 1—Restoring vision to the blind: The new age of implanted visual prostheses. Translational Vision Science & Technology. 2014;**3**:3-13. DOI: 10.1167/tvst.3.7.3

[92] da Cruz L, Fynes K, Georgiadis O, Kerby J, Luo YH, Ahmado A, et al. Phase 1 clinical study of an embryonic stem cell-derived retinal pigment epithelium patch in age-related macular degeneration. Nature Biotechnology. 2018;**36**:328-337. DOI: 10.1038/nbt.4114

[93] MacLaren RE, Groppe M, Barnard AR, Cottriall CL, Tolmachova T, Seymour L, et al. Retinal gene therapy in patients with choroideremia: Initial findings from a phase 1/2 clinical trial. Lancet. 2014;**383**:1129-1137. DOI: 10.1016/S0140-6736(13)62117-0

[94] Marc R, Pfeiffer R, Jones B. Retinal prosthetics, optogenetics, and chemical photoswitches. ACS Chemical Neuroscience. 2014;**5**:895-901. DOI: 10.1021/cn5001233

[95] Simunovic MP, Shen W, Lin JY, Protti DA, Lisowski L, Gillies MC. Optogenetic approaches to vision restoration. Experimental Eye Research. 2019;**178**:15-26

[96] Fenno L, Yizhar O, Deisseroth K. The development and application of optogenetics. Annual Review of Neuroscience. 2011;**34**:389-412. DOI: 10.1146/annurev-neuro-061010-113817

[97] Busskamp V, Picaud S, Sahel J-A, Roska B. Optogenetic therapy for retinitis pigmentosa. Gene Therapy. 2012;**19**:169-175. DOI: 10.1038/gt.2011.155

[98] Sengupta A, Chaffiol A, Macé E, Caplette R, Desrosiers M, Lampič M, et al. Red-shifted channelrhodopsin stimulation restores light responses in blind mice, macaque retina, and human retina. EMBO Molecular Medicine. 2016;**8**:1248-1264. DOI: 10.15252/emmm.201505699

[99] Chaffiol A, Caplette R, Jaillard C, Brazhnikova E, Desrosiers M, Dubus E, et al. A new promoter allows optogenetic vision restoration with enhanced sensitivity in macaque retina. Molecular Therapy. 2017;**25**:2546-2560. DOI: 10.1016/j.ymthe.2017.07.011

[100] Chuong AS, Miri ML, Busskamp V, Matthews GAC, Acker LC, Sørensen AT, et al. Noninvasive Optical Inhibition with a Red-Shifted Microbial Rhodopsin. Vol. 17. Nature Publishing Group; 2014. DOI: 10.1038/nn.3752

Chapter 7

Optimization of Maxillofacial Prosthesis

Faraedon M. Zardawi and Kaida Xiao

Abstract

Today, both additive manufacturing (3D image technology and 3D printing) had been developed dramatically and involved virtually in all fields of medicine and surgery. It has been widely applied in surgical and prosthetic reconstruction of the craniofacial defects. The aim of this chapter is to characterize and assess the mechanical and optical properties of 3D colored printed soft tissue facial prostheses produced by Z-Corp-Z510 and infiltrated with Sil-25 maxillofacial silicone polymers. Mechanical properties assessed according to ASTM specifications for tensile strength, tear strength, hardness and percentage elongation. Furthermore depth of infiltration plus quality of infiltration was assessed. Scanning electron microscopy SEM was applied for this purpose to determine the characteristic of interaction and incorporation between the starch powder particles and the silicone polymers. Finally, method of color reproduction and evaluation for the printed prostheses are recommended.

Keywords: maxillofacial, anaplastology, rapid prototyping and facial prostheses, skin color

1. Introduction

Anaplastology is a multidisciplinary branch of medicine that deals with artificial reconstruction of a disfigured, absent or anatomically malformed part of the face or body by fabricating a customized facial or somatic prosthesis for the patient [1]. The prostheses provide descriptive evidence for steps of fabrication of these devices, including location, retention, support, time, materials, and form [2, 3]. Prostheses are artificial devices which either implanted or attached to the body to replace or restore a body part that might be congenitally missing or might have been lost due to tumor ablation or external trauma [4]. Facial disfiguration is considered a challenge for the patient; as it negatively interferes with the patient's self-image and ability coexist in a normal social life. Although the prosthesis is well appreciated by the patients, however, in many instances it does not restore function totally [1, 5]. Surgery can repair small defects, whereas, large defects could not be repaired surgically [6], Hence, prosthetic rehabilitation is frequently applied. This depends on a variety of factors including patient's age and systemic condition, size and site of the defect, patient's satisfaction and cost factors [7–9]. For example, an old patient with poor systemic health is not a good candidate for surgery, on the other hand, an impaired vision or a poor manual dexterity patient is not a good candidate for prosthesis as he will not be able to maintain the prosthesis properly.

Defects in the craniofacial region mostly lead to severe depression, even in some instances to self-isolation and rejection of life, hence, surgical reconstruction and/or prosthetic devises will be an insistent demand for a patient with facial disfiguration [10]. Esthetically appropriate Prosthetic rehabilitation of the patient is rather challenging requires multidisciplinary team for comprehensive care and optimal cost treatment functional and esthetic outcomes [11–14]. Oro-facial areas comprises a variety of vital and important structures, every so often surgical management of cancer in this region predominantly with widespread cancerous lesion require extensive removal of tissue—the cancerous lesion and part from the normal tissue around the lesion as a protective measure of surgical management of cancer. As a result of this aggressive surgical procedure many vital functions would be impaired such as esthetics, phonetics, mastication and vision. In these cases an extensive defect would be left behind that would most probably not be reconstructed surgically, alternatively prosthetic rehabilitation will be performed to improve patient's esthetics/function [15, 16]. Prosthetic rehabilitation of these patient provides comfort to the patients, improves their confidence and self-esteem. High level of satisfaction was recorded among patients wearing facial prostheses [17]. They experienced much better quality of life after wearing facial prostheses [16, 18].

The fabrication protocol of facial prostheses involves several intricate steps as described by many authors [19–21] including taking an impression or impressions, obtaining an accurate stone cast in order to carve an accurate wax model for the defect on that cast. The wax model then checked on the patient and transferred to the final material, which is mostly be a silicone polymers by process of flasking and deflasking after adding the basic skin color. Ultimate color matching is accomplished by adding extrinsic colors at the time of fitting and delivery.

Method of fabrication that is applied currently has shown several limitations. These are primarily related to the fabrication protocol, high technical expertise required, time, effort, cost plus retention and esthetic problems. These limitations make access to global patient's community almost denied, only a small number of these patients can get access to this sophisticated device, those who can afford the high cost of the prosthesis, whereas, people at the other poor global regions such as Africa and India they cannot easily obtain a good prosthesis.

In recent years, both additive manufacturing (also known as 3D printing) and 3D image technology had been developed dramatically and becomes more and more popular in medical science under the term of medical rapid prototyping (MRP). Medical Rapid prototyping was first described by Mankowich et al. in 1990 for imaging and producing anatomically accurate human parts models by rapid prototyping methods [22]. MRP then started to grow more and more to involve a wide range and fields in medicine including tissue engineering, dental implantology, craniofacial surgery and reconstruction and orthopedics.

Many aspects of this brilliant technology have still not been entirely functional for maxillofacial surgical/prosthetic rehabilitation. This technology has not been fully incorporated in producing maxillofacial soft tissue prostheses. However, some articles and few case reports applied this technology in the manufacturing process as producing accurate wax models for ear and other parts of the face using 3D printing machines to be replicated by the silicone polymers [23–27]. They were able to produce highly accurate anatomical models of the missing parts, nevertheless, the entire procedure found to become more time consuming and much costly than if the prosthesis made by hand alone.

In our previous studies, an innovated method of fabrication of soft tissue facial prostheses using 3D color printing technology have been developed using Z-Corp

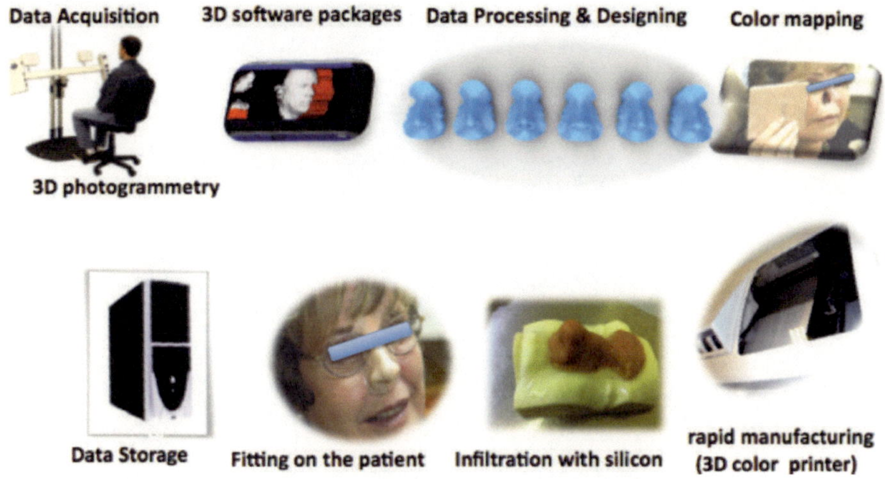

Figure 1.
An overview of rapid manufacturing technology applied to fabricate soft tissue facial prostheses.

printer, printing in starch as a powder and colored ink as a water based binder, printing process based on computer aided design and manufacture CAD/CAM [28–30]. **Figure 1** summarize the current project that starts with 3D Data acquisition instead of using a complicated multiple impression techniques, then processing these date in a 3D computer aided design—CAD package, building a virtual 3D model for the prosthesis, color mapping then the printing process accomplished using Z510-3D color printer. After printing the robot models infiltrated with elastomeric silicone in order to achieve skin texture and softness. Furthermore, data can be saved for future printing of further copies on demand.

With above protocol, there is huge potential to replace the conventional technology by the rapid manufacturing technology with saving both time and cost. However, some more factors affect quality of prostheses significantly, including mechanical properties, infiltration and degree of skin color reproduction. In this study, these factors are investigated and further developed. Results are described in following sections.

2. Mechanical properties

The mechanical properties of facial prostheses is very important since it directly related to durability of the prostheses. For 3D printing technology we proposed, a starch powder were used to print soft tissue prostheses by a Z-Corp Z510 3D printer and infiltrated using silicone polymers as the post processing. The mechanical properties of the composite produced by Z-Corp printer is tested here by comparing its' mechanical properties with object produced by silicone polymer using conventional technology [31].

Test models that were printed from starch by Z Corp 3D printer and infiltrated with maxillofacial silicone polymer—Sil-25 are shown in **Figure 2**.

Mechanical test for conventional technology is simulated using pure silicone polymers and used as control samples (**Figure 3**).

Pure silicone samples were designed according to ASTM specifications for tensile strength (Dumbbell-shaped specimens [32]), tear strength (Trouser-shaped specimens [33]), hardness test [34], and percentage elongation using solid work

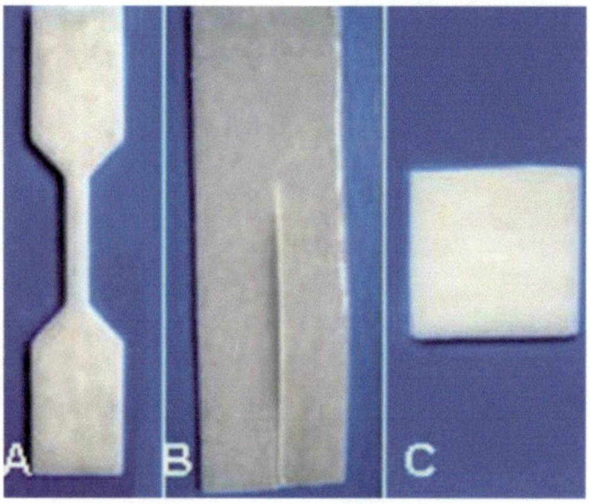

Figure 2.
Starch printed infiltrated silicone test samples for (A) dumbbell-shaped for tensile strength, (B) trouser-shaped for tear strength and (C) hardness test blocks.

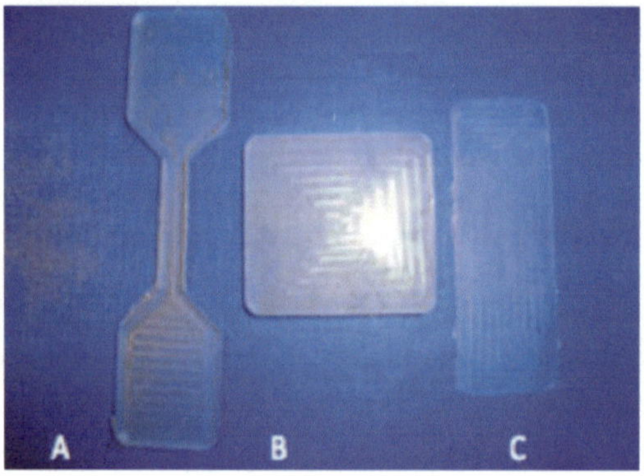

Figure 3.
Silicone polymers test samples for (A) dumbbell-shaped for tensile strength, (B) hardness test blocks and (C) trouser-shaped for tear strength.

2008 software for printing test samples and stainless steel molds were fabricated for the control samples (**Figure 4**).

Lloyd LRX tensile instrument applied to test tensile strength, tear strength and percentage elongation (**Figure 5**).

Shore Durometer Hardness Tester was applied to test the hardness of the 3D printed starch models infiltrated silicone polymers to be compared with pure silicone samples (**Figure 6**).

The collected data was analyzed using PASW statistics 18 to compare between the test group—3D printed samples and control group—pure silicone samples, Independent sample T test was utilized for the statistical analysis.

Table 1, Demonstrating the result of mechanical tests that reveals that test group—the 3D printed samples has significantly lower tensile, tear, and percentage elongation than control samples—pure silicone samples ($p < 0.05$). Whereas, a significant increase in the hardness of the printed samples compared to pure silicone samples ($p < 0.05$) as shown in **Table 1**.

The results indicated an increased hardness, and consequently the prostheses lose some flexibility, hardness is not the only issue that determine the flexibility, here the technology applied provide shell-like models and the prostheses built according to CAD/CAM is shell prosthesis showing high degree of flexibility than

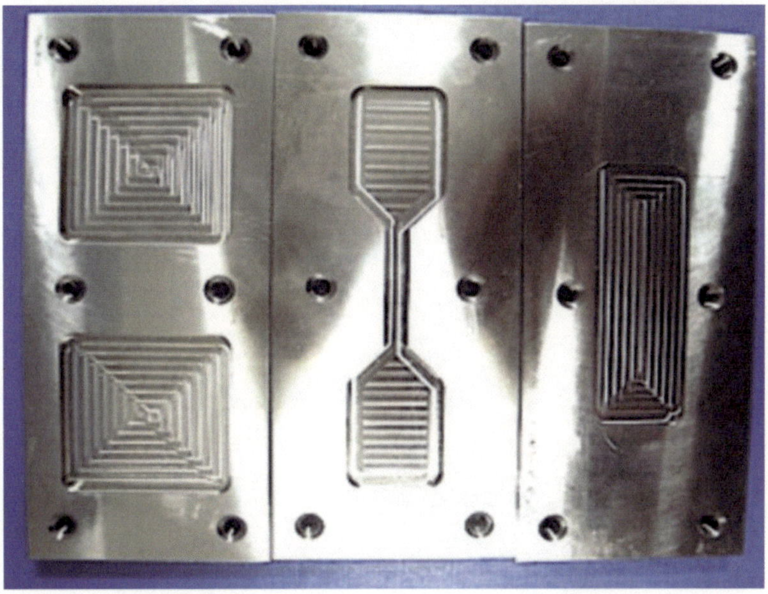

Figure 4.
Stainless steel molds for fabrication of control samples—pure silicone.

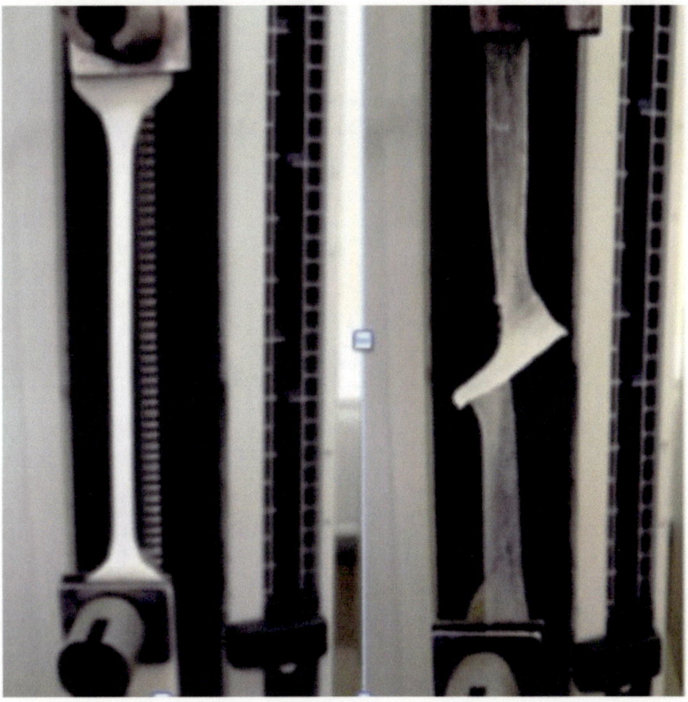

Figure 5.
Lloyd LRX tensile tester testing tensile and tear strength of the printed samples.

handmade prosthesis despite increased hardness of the printed prostheses compared to pure silicone prostheses as shown in **Figure 7**.

Lower values of tensile, tear strength and percentage elongation do not indicate a critical problem if the patient maintained and handled the prosthesis gently, as a matter of fact the prosthesis does not require a very high tensile or tear strength

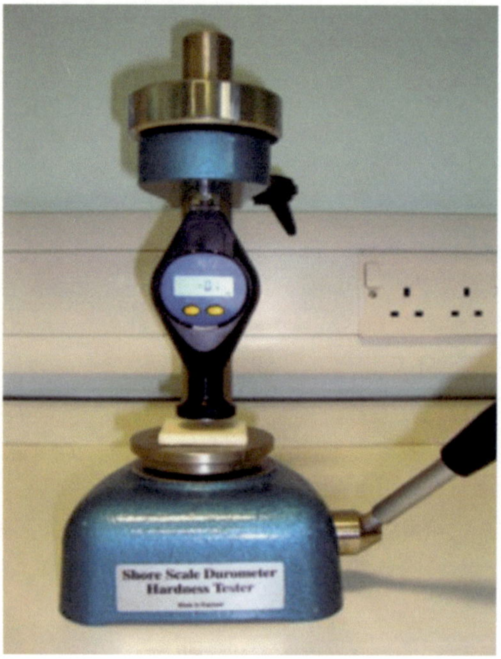

Figure 6.
Hardness tester testing hardness of the printed samples.

Sample	Tensile stress (PSI)	Tear stress (N/mm)	Hardness	Elongation (%)
Silicone (Convectional)				
Average	455.98	10.77	30.89	480.75
SD	32.20	2.60	0.71	84.40
Silicone infiltrated starch (3D printing)				
Average	170.45	8.02	62.80	221.46
SD	36.10	1.68	2.782	51.44

Table 1.
Comparing the mechanical properties of the printed models with pure silicone models.

unless the patient stretch his/or her prosthesis and handle it harshly. The patient should follow the instruction for maintenance cautiously so that to extend the prosthesis service life.

Investigations of mechanical properties (tensile, tear, hardness and percentage elongation) of the printed samples were significantly different from control samples. In this study the results of the mechanical tests performed on tensile strength, tear strength, the percentage of elongation and hardness for the printed samples were found to be significantly different from the control samples. According to results obtained from this study, no one can suggest that the manufactured prosthesis does not last long or not better than the handmade prosthesis, because the ideal properties have not been standardized yet in terms of the mechanical properties.

Variation in mechanical properties of the test samples compared with controlled samples—pure silicone samples could be perhaps due to amount of starch in the test material, as starch provides a scaffold for the silicone polymer when it is used by Z-Corp printer to produce three dimensional 3D facial prostheses. The starch

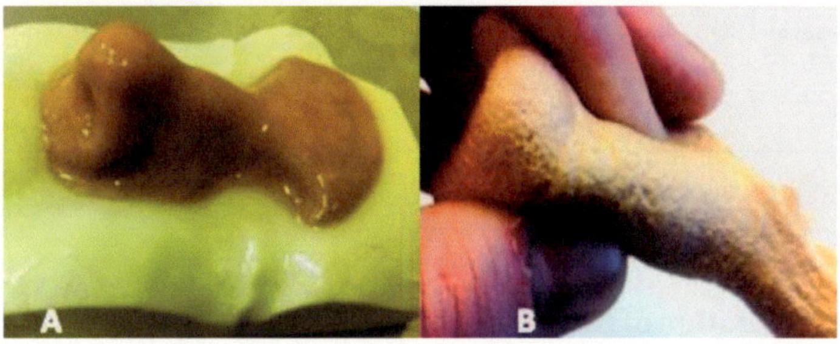

Figure 7.
(A) Method of infiltration leaving feather edged margin of the prosthesis. (B) Flexibility of printed prosthesis infiltrated silicone polymer.

acts as filler for the 3D printed prostheses, a filler when added to the silicone polymer may increases hardness, and reduces tensile and tear strength, of course that is depend on the type and amount of the filler [35, 36]. Therefore, it was necessary to measure the weight or volume ratio of silicone polymers—the infiltrate to starch—the filler. Furthermore, and in order to understand the variation in the mechanical properties and the general drawback in these properties it was necessary to investigate depth of penetration of the infiltrate (silicone polymers) inside the printed starch models the quality of this infiltration. Therefore, Proper protocols were designed for

1. Percentage of starch by weight within fully infiltrated models
2. Depth of infiltration inside printed starch models
3. Quality of infiltration and degree of coherence between the starch particles and the silicone polymers.

3. Infiltration

For 3D printing soft tissue prostheses process, the 3D printed starch models is infiltrated by silicone polymers in order to provide skin texture and required elasticity and softness. The infiltration process affects overall quality of prostheses and therefore investigated below in different aspects.

3.1 Silicone/powder ratio by weight

As the starch powder implicated in fabrication of 3 dimensional soft tissue prostheses, it was necessary to determine the average amount of this powder within the total weight of prosthesis and their percentages by weight in the final prosthesis. in this investigation, 8 printed blocks of the starch powder (45 × 45 × 4 mm) were produced by Z510 printer. The blocks weighed using a sensitive digital balance (Mettler AJ100). Then the samples infiltrated with Sil-25 maxillofacial silicone polymers according to infiltration protocol mentioned in the previous section (3 bars for 25 minutes left for 25 hours) final setting time. Then the infiltrated blocks weighed again and percentage of each component within an infiltrated block was determined. **Table 2** shows weight in gram, standard deviation and percentage of each component. The powder adds up to 40% of the total weight of the fully infiltrated blocks, whereas the silicone polymers comprising only 60%.

Weight in gram and SD		% By wight	
Starch	**Starch + Silicone pressure**	**Starch**	**Silicone pressure**
3.5 ± 0.04	8.50 ± 0.07	41.5%	58.5%

Table 2.
Percentage of silicone polymers and starch powder in fully infiltrated blocks.

3.2 Depth of infiltration of the silicone polymers into 3D printed facial prosthesis

As the printed starch models produced by the Z-Corp printer are solid and fragile, therefore, it was necessary to apply a specific protocol for infiltration of the silicone polymers into the printed models. For this purpose a set of 30 cubes measuring 20 × 20 × 20 mm were printed in starch, using Z-Corp (Z510) 3D printer, the starch cubes were infiltrated with Sil-25 maxillofacial silicone polymer under different conditions. One group served as control group, the cubes were infiltrated with Sil-25 maxillofacial silicone polymers, ratio (1–10) according to manufacturing standard. The cubes were then submerged in the polymer mixture and left under atmospheric air pressure at room temperature for a scheduled time, 5 minutes (n = 6), 10 minutes (n = 6), 15 minutes (n = 6), 20 minutes (n = 6) and 25 minutes (n = 6), and then left to set for 24 hours. The cubes then bisected with surgical blade No. 11. The inner part of the cube stained to color and highlight the non-infiltrated parts of the cubes in order to measure infiltration depth of the silicone polymers inside the cubes (**Figure 8**).

Three other groups were served as test groups, testing infiltration depth was repeated on 30 cubes measuring 20 × 20 × 20 mm for each test group, but in this group the cubes were placed in a pressure vessel under 1, 2 and 3 bars pressure for a similar time schedule, 5 minutes (n = 6), 10 minutes (n = 6), 15 minutes (n = 6), 20 minutes (n = 6) and 25 minutes (n = 6). After 24 hours the cubes were bisected and the inner part of the cubes colored then Traveling microscope (Mitutoyo TM) with X-Y coordinate, used to measure the infiltration depth, 12 measurements on each sectioned cube (**Figure 9**).

Result of this study is shown in **Figure 10** and **Table 3**, minimum depth of infiltration was detected under normal atmospheric pressure and room temperature, which was around 1 mm, this was slightly affected by length of time the cubes staid sank in the silicone polymers. Whereas, 2 and 3 bars pressure increased the infiltration depth of the silicone polymers significantly, which was also affected by length of time. Maximum infiltration depth was recorded for 3 bars pressure and at 25 minutes time. Results showed that pressure and time have significant effect on the depth of infiltration of the silicone polymers inside the powder cubes. Two ways ANOVA implied significant differences ($p < 0.05$) between the three groups of the current study, normal pressure, 2 and 3 bars pressure.

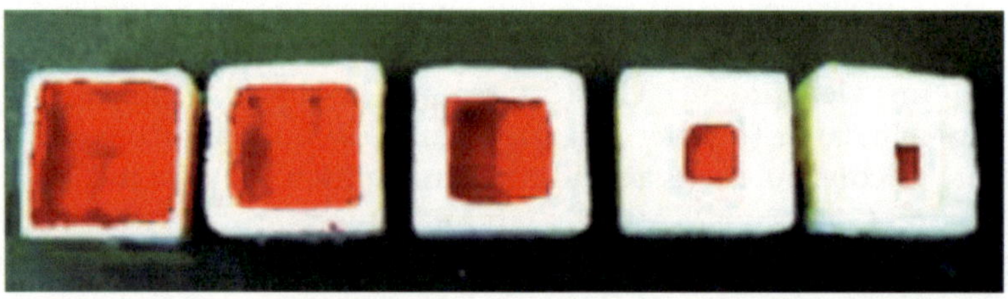

Figure 8.
Bisected cubes stained to identify the depth of infiltration of silicone polymers, the dye is taken up by the hydrophilic starch, whereas the infiltrated area is hydrophobic and does not take up the dye.

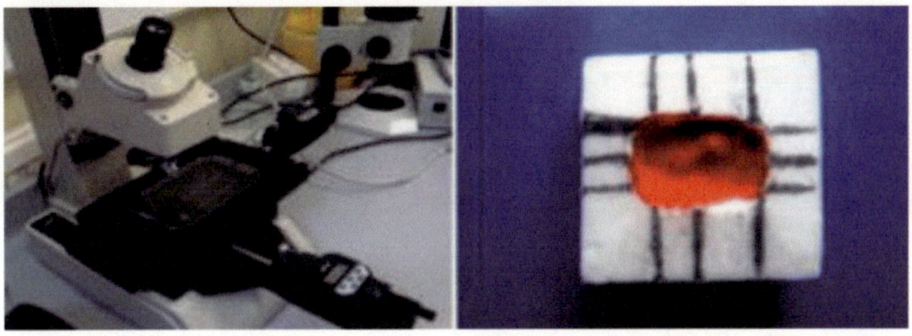

Figure 9.
Traveling microscope (Mitutoyo TM) with X-Y coordinate, used to measure the infiltration depth, 12 measurements on each sectioned cube.

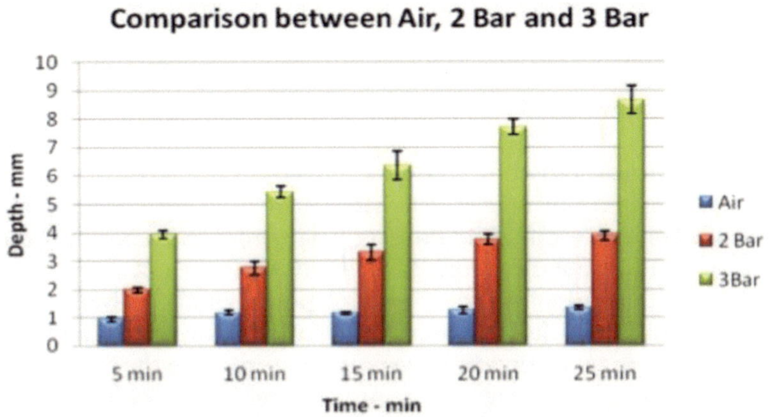

Figure 10.
Infiltration of Sil-25 under normal air, 2 and 3 bars pressure and 5-time schedule.

According to result obtained from this study, it can be concluded that infiltration depth of Sil-25 silicone polymers is significantly influenced by pressure applied. Under 3 bars and 25 minutes time, the infiltration depth recorded more than 8 mm from all sides, this would suggest that infiltration depth inside a prosthesis would be around 16 mm and reasonably this depth will be sufficient for soft tissue facial prostheses.

3.3 Quality of infiltration of the elastomer into 3D printed facial prosthesis

Evaluation of the infiltration quality of silicone polymers inside the 3D printed starch powder was required to characterize the interaction between the hydrophobic silicone polymers and the hydrophilic starch powder. It is acknowledged that the mechanical and optical properties of the 3D printed prostheses depend basically on material properties and characterization, which consequently determine the service life of the prostheses and determine its ability to resist the environmental factors such as UV from sunlight humidity, body secretion and weathering temperature. The previous section determined depth of infiltration of the infiltrate inside the printing powder, 8 mm penetration depth was achieved. However, we did not realize how consistent/homogeneous this infiltration was. Therefore, SEM was carried out to characterize an important aspect of 3D color printing facial prostheses and to detect any flaw in the structure of the composite that is utilized in fabrication of facial prostheses.

		Infiltration depth in (mm) and SD				
Infiltration time (minutes)		5 minutes	10 minutes	15 minutes	20 minutes	25 minutes
Silicone polymer	Pressure					
Sil-25	Air pressure	0.94 (0.08)	1.19 (0.01)	1.16 (0.05)	1.27 (0.13)	1.35 (0.08)
Sil-25	2 Bar	1.99 (0.10)	2.76 (0.23)	3.30 (0.28)	3.75 (0.19)	3.88 (0.17)
Sil-25	3 Bar	3.94 (0.15)	5.43 (0.20)	6.36 (0.51)	7.71 (0.27)	8.65 (0.49)

Table 3.
Infiltration depth of Sil-25 inside 3D printed starch blocks under different pressure and at different time schedule.

3.3.1 Slide preparation for SEM

Scanning Electron Microscopy SEM was applied for this purpose to prepare and obtain various samples of printed starch blocks infiltrated with two different maxillofacial silicone polymers (Sil25 and Promax 10) in order to examine the quality of the infiltration inside the starch printed blocks. SEM pictures of the printed blocks were compared with hand mixed of 40% starch powder and 60% Sil25 silicone polymers. Hand mixed blocks were prepared by mixing the starch and the silicone polymers for 1 minute to obtain a homogenous mixture, then the mixture poured into a 75 × 75 × 4 mm stainless steel mold, pressed and left for 24 hours in ambient temperature. Then slices from the three blocks were prepared using surgical blade number 11 and send for SEM to be examined with SEM of starch powder alone.

3.3.2 SEM interpretation

SEM analysis of the starch powder, 3D printed blocks infiltrated Sil-25 and Promax10 plus the hand mixed blocks are shown in **Figure 11**, the SEM of the powder and of the infiltrated powder blocks showed amorphous, non-crystalline shaped particles with different particle sizes varies from very small to relatively large particles. These particles appeared to be loosely arranged and randomly orientated with some spaces in between these particles and disorganized spreading of the starch powder within the silicone polymers leaving big gaps between the powder particles. Incorporation of starch powder with Sil-25 maxillofacial silicone and Promax10 under 3 bar pressure are seen in **Figure 11A** and **B**, showing almost similar distribution of the powder within the infiltrates. However, better incorporation and more homogenous distribution of starch particles within the silicone polymers in hand mixed of 40% powder incorporated into 60% infiltrate of silicone polymers by weight (**Figure 11C**). This could be attributed to the layer of binder on the outer surfaces of the printed blocks that might an obstacle for the infiltration process.

3.3.3 Final analysis of SEM

Figure 12 is a magnified SEM image (×707) of hand mixed starch powder and Sil-25 silicone polymers. Although at a lower magnification the sample apparently seems to be very properly infiltrated having smooth texture, however, under higher

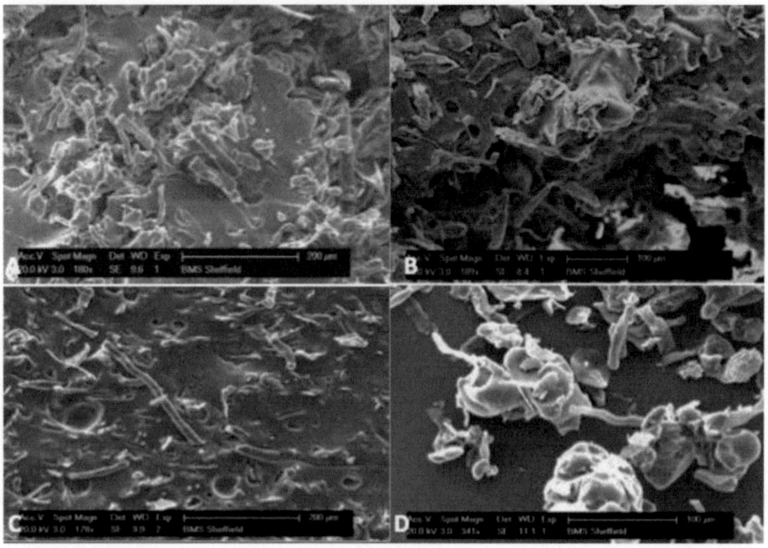

Figure 11.
SEM for (A) 3D printed starch block infiltrated Sil-25 SP (×180), (B) 3D printed starch block infiltrated Promax10 (×189), (C) hand mixed starch powder and Sil-25 SP (×178), (D) starch powder particles (×341).

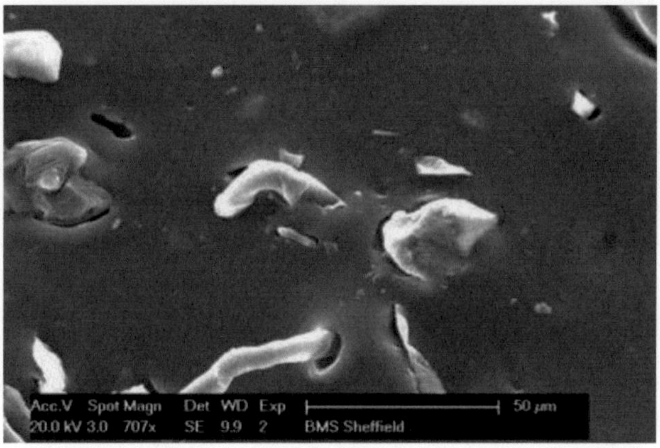

Figure 12.
SEM for Sil-25 hand mixed samples showing spaces around the starch particles (×707).

magnification the composite shows evidence of porosity and spaces between the powder particles and the silicone polymers within the composite. This phenomenon indicates lack of coherence and integrity between the hydrophobic silicone polymers and the hydrophilic starch powder, which, is related to the wettability and viscosity between silicone polymers that have low surface energy and strongly hydrophobic [37] and starch powder is hydrophilic in nature [38].

Furthermore SEM sections (**Figures 11C** and **12**) showing gaps and voids, which indicate tripping of air especially in central parts of the blocks under infiltration pressure. Lack of interaction and incorporation between the starch powder particles and the silicone polymers that are utilized by Z-Corp printer and employed for fabrication of soft tissue facial prostheses will influence the general properties and material's integrity, which my finally affect the durability of the prostheses. Therefore, it was necessary to test the mechanical properties of the 3D printed samples that are going to be used for fabrication of soft tissue facial prostheses.

4. Skin color reproduction

Skin color is vital for quality of facial prostheses. Previous research has focused on reproducing skin color and assess their color appearance difference under standard lighting conditions [39, 40]. The advent of new lighting technologies such as Halogen and LEDs generates new challenges for rendering skin on displays, in print, but most importantly, for synthetically generated skin prostheses, since ambient illumination can change the appearance of both natural and synthetic skin, but not necessarily in the same way [41]. Here skin appearance models not only need to take into account different ambient illuminations, but also the three-dimensionally geometry of the human face and differences in the methods for reconstruction—surgery, prosthetics or medical make-up/tattooing [42]. Therefore, to truly reproduce appearance of skin color under different illumination and objectively evaluate their color quality, follow steps are develop:

Step 1: Measurement of skin spectral reflectance of subject

The measurement of skin spectral reflectance would be affected by these various parameters, including the measurement instruments, measurement distance, measurement location, the instrument aperture size, the pressure applied to the skin by the instrument, as well as the gender and ethnic group [43]. Spectrophotometer is recommended for facial prostheses application, since it is independent of lighting applied and highly consistency [44].

Step 2: Develop spectral color profile for 3D camera

3D camera can be used to capture facial and body image. A spectral reflectance estimation need to conduct to transform camera RGB to spectral reflectance for each pixel of 3D image [45]. Spectral color database [46, 47]need to be used as training sample to obtain base function for spectral reflectance estimation.

Step 3: Develop spectral color profile for 3D printer

For 3D color printing, spectral color profile also needs to develop to transform spectral reflectance of human skin in each pixel of 3D image to printer CMYK value for color printing. Post printing processing also needs to conducted for infiltration process as described in previous section

Step 4: Color quality evaluation

To evaluate color quality of facial prostheses, the average CIELAB color difference (ΔEab) under several standard CIE illuminants needs to calculated. To test spectral reproduction, the root-mean-square error (RMSE) and goodness-of-fit coefficient (GFC) needs to apply [48].

5. Discussion

Drawback in the mechanical properties of the printed samples mostly attributed to the amount of starch (40%) and due to lack of coherence and integrity between the hydrophobic silicone polymers and the hydrophilic starch powder that form the scaffold for the test samples as Z Corp 3D printer utilizing starch powder for printing which led to draw back in the mechanical properties of the final product. Perhaps the prostheses will have a shorter service life than the conventional pure silicone prosthesis. However, printing several prostheses at time of printing could compensate the drawback in the mechanical properties. The technology applied enabled construction of several copies of the prostheses in a shorter time frame and at a lower cost than handmade silicone polymer prostheses. Another advantage of applying rapid prototyping is that producing the required thickness of the missing part that rendering a lightweight prosthesis, which is mostly valued by the patients (**Figure 13**).

Furthermore, designing a prosthesis by using 3D software package can also allow the anaplastologist to save the design and all patients data to utilize it for printing future copies of the prosthesis on the patients' demand and with only light modification in the design of the prosthesis if there is any tissue change at the site of the

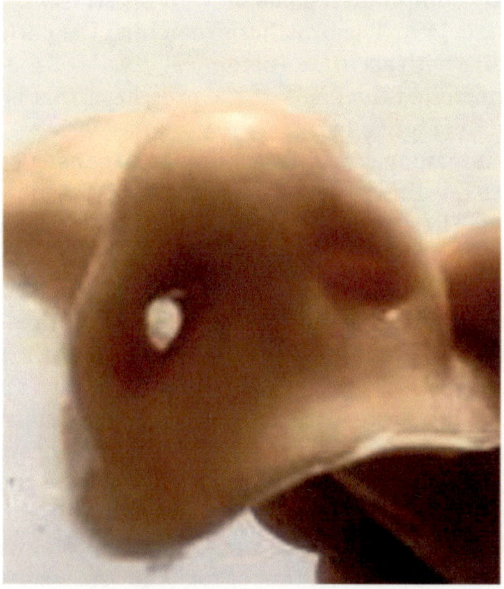

Figure 13.
3D printed nasal prosthesis showing nostril opened due to controlled thickness of the prosthesis.

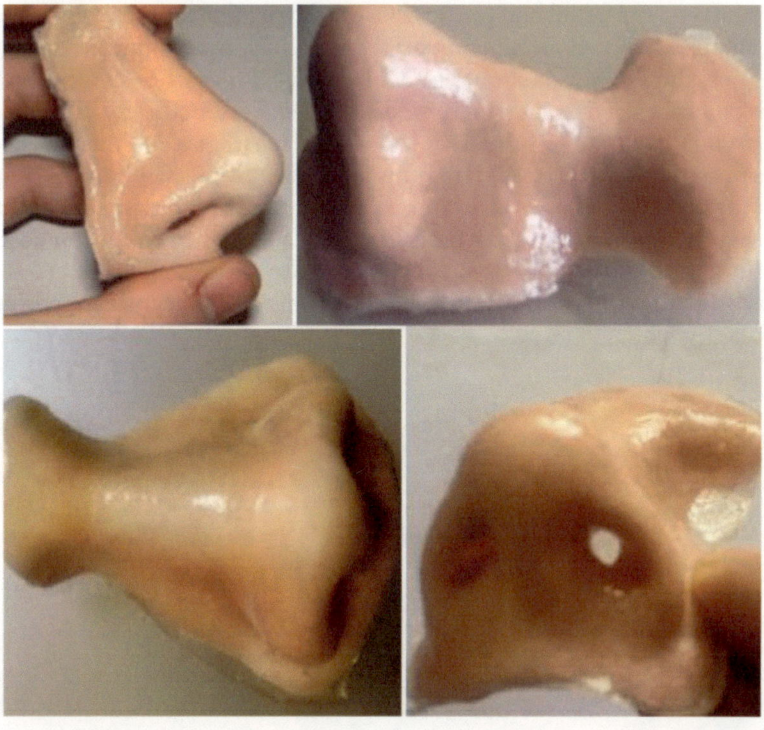

Figure 14.
Nasal prostheses produced by Z510-3D color printer.

defect [28]. Finally we believe that the many limitations of handmade prostheses regarding esthetics, high prosthesis cost, time, effort, hectic impression techniques and problems of retention plus high technical skill required for fabrication by anaplastologist could be generally reduced and consequently minimizing the social and psychological challenges that often-maxillofacial patients encountered in life.

At this stage, a fully computerized customized prosthesis is manufactured, using biocompatible materials [49]. The prosthesis matching the patient's skin color and having skin-like texture with accurate anatomical details of the patient, possessing a light weight with controlled thickness of the prosthesis that is well appreciated by the patients as shown in (**Figure 14**).

Despite the many advantages of this technology in constructing soft tissue facial prostheses, there were few limitations compared to handmade—conventional method of fabrication. These limitations were related to the mechanical properties of the final product [50]. The mechanical tests shows drawback in the mechanical properties, however, it is hard to judge how poorly that will affect the prosthesis on the patient; the only real way of testing mechanical and optical durability is when the prostheses test on the patients during the service life of the prosthesis. As the project was at the experimental stage of development it wasn't possible to perform these tests on patients [28]. More work should be done to determine how long the prostheses would last. So far it is obvious that the prostheses done need to be replaced regularly. Further investigations should be done on the printing materials in order to improve the mechanical properties and durability of the prostheses and to achieve optimal advantages of time compression technology and rapid prototyping for simple, full automated fabrication of facial prostheses.

6. Conclusion

Color matched maxillofacial prosthesis was fabricated using Z-Corp 510 color printer utilizing starch based biocompatible materials. According to the mechanical properties, the prosthesis should be replaced in a range of 6–12 months. The prosthesis could be used as interim prosthesis special after surgery while the patient is going through healing period. Furthermore the prosthesis could be used as definitive prostheses by compensating the draw back in the mechanical properties by taking the great advantages of this great technology that having the ability of printing several copies of the prosthesis at the time of printing at lower cost and rapid manufacturing of anatomically more accurate parts compared to handmade prostheses and applying more comfortable methods of data capturing, designing and manufacturing.

Author details

Faraedon M. Zardawi[1] and Kaida Xiao[2]*

1 University of Sulaymaniyah, Iraq

2 University of Leeds, United Kingdom

*Address all correspondence to: k.xiao1@leeds.ac.uk

References

[1] Karthikeyan I. A review on prosthetic rehabilitation of maxillofacial region. Anaplastology. 2014;**3**:125

[2] Glossary. The glossary of prosthodontic terms. The Journal of Prosthetic Dentistry. 2005;**94**:10-92

[3] Worthington P, Brånemark PI. Advanced Osseointegration Surgery: Applications in the Maxillofacial Region. Quintessence Pub Co.; 1992

[4] Poduval J. Branemark ear and nose prosthesis. International Journal of Medical Sciences and Biotechnology. 2013;**1**:1-16

[5] Gotay C, Moore T. Assessing quality of life in head and neck cancer. Quality of Life Research. 1992;**1**(1):5-17

[6] Van der Lei B et al. Nasal reconstruction with an expanded forehead flap after oncological ablation: Results, complications and a review of the English language literature. Faces. 1996;**3**:139-146

[7] Sencimen M, Gulses A. Implant retained auricular prostheses. In: Current Concepts in Plastic Surgery. InTech; 2012

[8] Brown KE. Clinical considerations improving obturator treatment. Journal of Prosthetic Dentistry. 1970;**24**(4):461-466

[9] Desjardins RP. Obturator prosthesis design for acquired maxillary defects. Journal of Prosthetic Dentistry. 1978;**39**(4):424-435

[10] Federspil P, Federspil P. Prosthetic management of craniofacial defects. Hals-Nasen-Ohrenheilkunde. 1998;**46**(6):569-578

[11] Dingman C, Hegedus PD, Likes C, McDowell P, McCarthy E, Zwilling C. A coordinated, multidisciplinary approach to caring for the patient with head and neck cancer. The Journal of Supportive Oncology. 2008;**6**(3):125-131

[12] Hubálková H, Holakovský J, Brázda F, Diblík P, Mazánek J. Team approach in treatment of extensive maxillofacial defects—Five case report serie. Prague Medical Report. 2010;**111**(2):148-157

[13] Clarke LK. Rehabilitation for the head and neck cancer patient. Oncology-Williston Park Then Huntington. 1998;**12**:81-90

[14] Lemon JC, Kiat-amnuay S, Gettleman L, Martin JW, Chambers MS. Facial prosthetic rehabilitation: Preprosthetic surgical techniques and biomaterials. Current Opinion in Otolaryngology & Head and Neck Surgery. 2005;**13**(4):255-262

[15] Leonardi A, Buonaccorsi S, Pellacchia V, Moricca LM, Indrizzi E, Fini G. Maxillofacial prosthetic rehabilitation using extraoral implants. The Journal of Craniofacial Surgery. 2008;**19**(2):398-405

[16] Mantri S, Khan Z. Prosthodontic rehabilitation of acquired maxillofacial defects. In: Head and Neck Cancer. InTech; 2012

[17] Goiato MC, Pesqueira AA, Ramos da Silva C, Gennari Filho H, Micheline Dos Santos D. Patient satisfaction with maxillofacial prosthesis. Literature review. Journal of Plastic, Reconstructive & Aesthetic Surgery. 2009;**62**(2):175-180

[18] Lowental U, Sela M. Evaluating cosmetic results in maxillofacial prosthetics. Journal of Prosthetic Dentistry. 1982;**48**(5):567-570

[19] Wang R. Preoperative auricular wax pattern duplication for surgical template

fabrication. The Journal of Prosthetic Dentistry. 1999;**81**(5):634-637

[20] Marion LR, Rothenbergerb SL, Minsley GE. A method of fabrication of a facial prosthesis that improves retention and durability: A clinical report. Journal of Prosthetic Dentistry. 1997;**77**(5):457-460

[21] Al Mardini M, Ercoli C, Graser GN. A technique to produce a mirror-image wax pattern of an ear using rapid prototyping technology. The Journal of Prosthetic Dentistry. 2005;**94**(2):195-198

[22] Mankovich NJ, Cheeseman AM, Stoker NG. The display of three-dimensional anatomy with stereolithographic models. Journal of Digital Imaging. 1990;**3**(3):200-203

[23] Chen LH, Tsutsumi S, Iizuka T. A CAD/CAM technique for fabricating facial prostheses: A preliminary report. The International Journal of Prosthodontics. 1997;**10**(5):467-472

[24] Bibb R, Freeman P, Brown R, Sugar A, Evans P, Bocca A. An investigation of three-dimensional scanning of human body surfaces and its use in the design and manufacture of prostheses. Proceedings of the Institution of Mechanical Engineers. Part H. 2000;**214**(6):589-594

[25] Subburaj K, Nair C, Rajesh S, Meshram SM, Ravi B. Rapid development of auricular prosthesis using CAD and rapid prototyping technologies. International Journal of Oral and Maxillofacial Surgery. 2007;**36**(10):938-943

[26] Ciocca L, Scotti R. CAD-CAM generated ear cast by means of a laser scanner and rapid prototyping machine. The Journal of Prosthetic Dentistry. 2004;**92**(6):591-595

[27] Cheah CM, Chua CK, Tan KH. Integration of laser surface digitizing with CAD/CAM techniques for developing facial prostheses. Part 2: Development of molding techniques for casting prosthetic parts. The International Journal of Prosthodontics. 2003;**16**(5):543-548

[28] Zardawi FM. Characterisation of Implant Supported Soft Tissue Prostheses Produced with 3D Color Printing Technology [thesis]. University of Sheffield; 2013

[29] Xiao K, Zardawi F, van Noort R, Yates JM. Developing a 3D color image reproduction system for additive manufacturing of facial prostheses. The International Journal of Advanced Manufacturing Technology. 2014;**70**(9-12):2043-2049

[30] Xiao K, Wuerger S, Mostafa F, Sohaib A, Yates JM. Color image reproduction for 3D printing facial prostheses. In: Shishkovsky IV, editor. New Trends in 3D Printing. InTech; 2016. pp. 89-109

[31] Lai JH, Wang LL, Ko CC, DeLong RL, Hodges JS. New organosilicon maxillofacial prosthetic materials. Dental Materials. 2002;**18**(3):281-286

[32] ASTM-D412. D412 standard test methods for rubber properties in tension. In: Annual Book of ASTM Standards. Philadelphia: ASTM Designation: American Society for Testing and Materials; 1981

[33] ASTM-D624. ASTM designation: D624 standard test method for rubber property-tear resistance. In: Annual Book of ASTM Standards. Philadelphia; 1981. p. 37

[34] ASTM D 2240, Standard test method for rubber property-Durometer hardness. Figure S. left column shows yisual surbet'degradation of the ont'-compont'nt urethane after (top to bottom), 2000. 18

[35] Ciocca L, Fantini M, De Crescenzio F, Persiani F, Scotti R. New protocol for construction of eyeglasses-supported provisional nasal prosthesis using CAD/CAM techniques. Journal of Rehabilitation Research and Development. 2010;**47**(7):595-604

[36] Aziz T, Waters M, Jagger R. Analysis of the properties of silicone rubber maxillofacial prosthetic materials. Journal of Dentistry. 2003;**31**(1):67-74

[37] Waters MG, Jagger RG, Polyzois GL. Wettability of silicone rubber maxillofacial prosthetic materials. The Journal of Prosthetic Dentistry. 1999;**81**:439-443

[38] Jayasekara R, Harding I, Bowater I, Christie GBY, Lonergan GT. Preparation, surface modification and characterisation of solution cast starch PVA blended films. Polymer Testing. 2004;**23**(1):17-27

[39] Xiao K, Zardawi F, van Noort R, Yates JM. Color reproduction for advanced manufacture of soft tissue prostheses. Journal of Dentistry. 2013;**41**:e15-e23

[40] Paravina RD, Majkic G, Del Mar Perez M, Kiat-amnuay S. Color difference thresholds of maxillofacial skin replications. Journal of Prosthodontics. 2009;**18**:618-625

[41] Melgosa M, Richard N, Fernández-Maloigne C, Xiao K, de Clermont-Gallerande H, Jost-Boissard S, et al. Color differences in Caucasian and oriental women's faces illuminated by white light-emitting diode sources. International Journal of Cosmetic Science. 2018;**40**(3):244-255

[42] Sohaib A, Amano K, Xiao K, Yates JM, Whitford C, Wuerger S. Color quality of facial prostheses in additive manufacturing. International Journal of Advanced Manufacturing Technology. 2018;**96**(1-4):881-894

[43] Wang M, Xiao K, Luo MR, Pointer M, Cheung V, Wuerger S. An investigation into the variability of skin color measurements. Color Research and Application. 2018;**43**(4):458-470

[44] Wang Y, Luo MR, Wang M, Xiao K, Pointer M. Spectrophotometric measurement of human skin color. Color Research and Application. 2017;**42**(6):764-774

[45] Xiao K, Zhu Y, Li C, Connah D, Yates JM, Wuerger S. Improved method for skin reflectance reconstruction from camera images. Optics Express. 2016;**24**(13):14934-14950

[46] Xiao K, Yates JM, Zardawi F, Sueeprasan S, Liao N, Gill L, et al. Characterising the variations in ethnic skin colors: A new calibrated data base for human skin. Skin Research and Technology. 2017;**23**(1):21-29

[47] Xiao K, Liao N, Zardawi F, Liu H, Noort RV, Yang Z, et al. Investigation of Chinese skin color and appearance for skin color reproduction. Chinese Optics Letters. 2012;**10**(8):083301-083305

[48] Liang J, Xiao K, Pointer M, Wan X, Li C. Spectra estimation from raw camera responses based on adaptive local-weighted linear regression. Optics Express. 2019;**27**(4):5165-5180

[49] Zardawi FM, Yadev N, Noort R, Yates JM. In-vitro evaluation of the cytotoxicity of binders and powder used in 3D color printing of maxillofacial soft tissue prostheses. IOSR Journal of Dental and Medical Sciences. 2015;**14**(8):59-64

[50] Zardawi FM, Xiao K, Noort R, Yates JM. Mechanical properties of 3D printed facial prostheses compared to handmade silicone polymer prostheses. European Scientific Journal, ESJ. 2015;**11**(12):1-11